Gender and the Social Construction of Illness

THE GENDER LENS SERIES

Series Editors

Judith A. Howard
University of Washington

Barbara Risman
North Carolina State University

Joey Sprague
University of Kansas

The Gender Lens Series has been conceptualized as a way of encouraging the development of a sociological understanding of gender. A "gender lens" means working to make gender visible in social phenomena; asking if, how, and why social processes, standards, and opportunities differ systematically for women and men. It also means recognizing that gender inequality is inextricably braided with other systems of inequality. The Gender Lens series is committed to social change directed toward eradicating these inequalities. Originally published by Sage Publications and Pine Forge Press, all Gender Lens books are now available from AltaMira Press.

BOOKS IN THE SERIES

Yen Le Espiritu, *Asian American Women and Men: Labor, Laws, and Love*

Judith A. Howard and Jocelyn A. Hollander, *Gendered Situations, Gendered Selves: A Gender Lens on Social Psychology*

Michael A. Messner, *Politics of Masculinities: Men in Movements*

Judith Lorber and Lisa Jean Moore, *Gender and the Social Construction of Illness*, Second Edition

Scott Coltrane, *Gender and Families*

Myra Marx Ferree, Judith Lorber, and Beth B. Hess, editors, *Revisioning Gender*

Pepper Schwartz and Virginia Rutter, *The Gender of Sexuality: Exploring Sexual Possibilities*

Francesca M. Cancian and Stacey J. Oliker, *Caring and Gender*

M. Bahati Kuumba, *Gender and Social Movements*

Toni M. Calasanti and Kathleen F. Slevin, *Gender, Social Inequalities, and Aging*

Gender and the Social Construction of Illness

Second Edition

Judith Lorber and Lisa Jean Moore

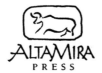

ALTAMIRA
PRESS

A Division of
ROWMAN & LITTLEFIELD PUBLISHERS, INC.
Lanham • Boulder • New York • Toronto • Plymouth, UK

ALTAMIRA PRESS
A division of Rowman & Littlefield Publishers, Inc.
A wholly owned subsidary of The Rowman & Littlefield Publishing Group, Inc
4501 Forbes Boulevard, Suite 200
Lanham, MD 20706
www.altamirapress.com

Estover Road
Plymouth PL6 7PY
United Kingdom

British Library Cataloguing in Publication Information Available

Library of Congress Cataloging-in-Publication Data

Lorber, Judith.
    Gender and the social construction of illness / Judith Lorber and Lisa Jean Moore.—
2nd ed.
      p. cm.—(The gender lens series)
    Includes bibliographical references and index.
    ISBN: 978-0-7591-0238-5
    1. Social medicine. 2. Women—Health and hygiene. 3. Sexism in medicine. I. Moore,
Lisa Jean, 1967– II. Title. III. Gender lens.

    RA418 .L67 2002
    306.461—dc21

                           2002003798

Printed in the United States of America

♾™ The paper used in this publication meets the minimum requirements of American National Standard for Information Sciences—Permanence of Paper for Printed Library Materials, ANSI/NISO Z39.48–1992.

For Lorrie and Phyllis,
who have gone through life with Judith

For Grace and Georgia,
who begin life with Lisa

CONTENTS

The current volume is the second edition of *Gender and the Social Construction of Illness*. Judith Lorber and Lisa Jean Moore present a gendered analysis of health, illness, and medical care. This volume is thoroughly updated, and adds chapters on disability and genital surgery. Judith Lorber and Lisa Jean Moore use familiar concepts in medical sociology reconceptualized through a gender lens. Like the first edition, the current volume addresses two basic issues. First, the authors pay critical attention to the social aspects of the experience of physical illness and resultant medical care. This involves attention to how gender, race, class, ethnicity, and culture influence the experience of symptoms and how such symptoms are treated by the medical establishment. Second, the authors use a gender lens to critically examine the social construction of the knowledge base and underlying assumptions about illness. They critique the way questions are asked and research priorities set.

Although medical sociologists have addressed these issues in the past, they have usually done so without a gender lens. For medical sociologists, gender has meant women—first, patients and nurses, and then doctors. When medical sociologists have added women to research it has usually meant comparing women's and men's sickness and death rates, differences in behavior and in treatment as patients, behaviors as doctors, and so on. But much of the analysis of the social construction of medical knowledge and beliefs did not incorporate a concern with the social construction of gender.

For feminists who study health and illness, attention to gender has meant concern with the status of women and men in the social order. Feminists have asked why, how, and by whom such normal physiological events as menstruation and menopause have been turned into illnesses and consequently into social problems. They have looked at the gendered dimensions of the hierarchy of medical occupations and what happens when men are nurses and women are doctors. Feminists have also questioned the objectivity and neutrality of scientific findings that come out of a professional world dominated by men.

In this volume, Judith Lorber and Lisa Jean Moore weave together medical, sociological, and feminist concerns as they take a gender lens on health, illness, and medicine. Lorber and Moore show how gender is an integral part of the transformation of physiology—rates of illness and longevity—and provide data for the proposition that these are the results of social statuses—race, class, and gender. Premenstrual tension and menopause are discussed at length as examples of the processes by which normal physiological female phenomena become illnesses that denigrate women's social status. Lorber and Moore provide an in-depth look at the current AIDS epidemic. The book ends with a proposal for leveling the hierarchies and inequalities in medicine through feminist health care practices and suggests that this would be beneficial for men as well as for women.

We hope this book, and others in the Gender Lens series, will help the reader develop her or his own "gender lens" to better and more accurately understand our social environments. As sociologists, we believe that an accurate understanding of inequality is a prerequisite for effective social change.

Judith Howard
Barbara Risman
Joey Sprague
Gender Lens Series Editors

ACKNOWLEDGMENTS

Thanks go to Mitch Allen for getting both editions of this book going, and to the editors of the Gender Lens series—Judy Howard, Barbara Risman, Mary Romero, and Joey Sprague—for their encouragement and advice. For the first edition, Elianne Riska suggested the theoretical work on the social construction of the body; Edward J. Farrell Jr. supplied life-expectancy statistics; and Joyce Wallace and Brenda Seals reviewed the chapter on AIDS. Judi Addelston and the reference librarians at the Mina Reese CUNY Graduate School Library provided indispensable literature searches for the first edition. To them go Judith's thanks.

For the second edition, we would both like to thank Patricia Clough for suggesting our collaboration and Barbara Risman for critiquing the entire manuscript. Thanks also go to Robyn Mierzwa for thorough and meticulous readings.

Chapter 3, "Hierarchies in Health Care," is adapted from Judith Lorber, "Gender Hierarchies in the Health Professions," in *Gender Mosaics: Social Perspectives*, edited by Dana Vannoy, Roxbury, 2001. Chapter 4, "Gender and Disability," is adapted from Judith Lorber, "Gender Contradictions and Status Dilemmas in Disability," in *Expanding the Scope of Social Science Research on Disability*, edited by Sharon N. Barnatt and Barbara M. Altman, JAI Press, 2000.

Even though we had completed the first draft of this second edition before September 11, 2001, we feel it is important to acknowledge the connection we saw between what we had written and the World Trade Center, Pentagon, and Pennsylvania attacks, and the subsequent anthrax contaminations, illnesses, and deaths. Living in New York City, our experiences were local, but we were constantly reminded of the global effects and the vulnerability of national borders. The rhetoric of epidemics, carriers, and contagion, the different impacts on women and men, the social class and racial ethnic implications, all replicated much of what is contained in this book. A long-term global perspective tells us that war, fear of terrorism, economic sanctions and embargoes, and institutionalized racism and oppression will continue to affect the lives, health, and bodies of people throughout the world. We hope that the feminist perspective on illness and death that is the framework of this book will help illuminate the trajectory of events that both preceded and follow that fateful Tuesday.

CHAPTER 1

Gender and the Social Construction of Illness: Overview

It has been assumed that anything and everything worth understanding can be explained or interpreted within the assumptions of modern science. Yet there is another world hidden from the consciousness of science—the world of emotions, feelings, political values; of the individual and collective unconscious; of social and historical particularity.... Part of the project of feminism is to reveal the relationship between these two worlds—how each shapes and forms the other. (Harding 1986, 245)

Illness is not just a physical state; it is a social phenomenon. Different cultures consider some physical states "illness" that others consider "normal." Westerners usually consider physical health as a state in which people can do what they have to do and want to do, and illness as something that disturbs the physiological equilibrium of the body. But what we actually experience as illness is a disturbance of our social lives so that we cannot go about our usual pursuits, a situation which may or may not be the result of actual bodily dysfunctioning. The perception that something is wrong and the guesses as to the cause are always experienced in a social context. Thus, a homemaker in a poor community, when asked to define illness, said:

> I wish I really knew what you meant about being sick. Sometimes I felt so bad I could curl up and die, but had to go on because the kids had to be taken care of, and besides, we didn't have the money to spend for the

doctor—how could I be sick? . . . How do you know when you're sick, anyway? Some people can go to bed almost any time with anything, but most of us can't be sick—even when we need to be. (Koos 1954, 30)

In every society, the symptoms, pains, and weaknesses considered "being sick" are shaped by cultural and moral values, experienced through interaction with members of one's immediate social circle and visits to health care professionals and influenced by beliefs about health and illness. The result is a transformation of physiological symptoms into illnesses with labels (diagnoses) and the people who have them into "patients." This transformation is heavily influenced by power differences and moral judgments. Not all patients are equal—gender, racial ethnic category, social class, physical ability, sexual orientation, and type of illness produce differences in social worth. Not all health care workers are equal, either—their place in the professional hierarchy determines their power to set research priorities, determine treatment modes, and produce what is considered legitimate medical knowledge.

In Western societies, the culture and language of illness and medical knowledge comes from science—"medical science" is the way we talk about what health care providers know and do. The *biomedical model* of illness assumes that disease is a deviation from normal physiological functioning, that diseases have specific causes that can be located in the ill person's body, that illnesses have the same symptoms and outcome in any social situation, and that medicine is a socially neutral application of scientific research to individual cases (Mishler 1981). Critics of this model have shown that what is normal depends on who is being compared to whom, that many diseases have social and environmental causes, that illness rates and severity vary from place to place, and that the values underlying medical research, practice, theories, and knowledge are deeply biased by the practice situations and the social characteristics of the dominant group of medical professionals—physicians.[1]

Critical medical sociologists provided ample evidence of racial and class biases in Western medicine, and feminists added gender to the list.[2] They argued that medical norms were based on White, middle-class men's bodies, and that physicians did not take women's daily lives into account when considering the causes of diseases or prescribing treatment. Most crucial, they challenged scientific claims to universality. How could medical science be trusted, they asked, when so few women were scientists, when the diseases that killed men were the first priority in research, when women were not included in clinical trials, and when women's bodies and experiences were ignored as data? The impact of the feminist critique of biomedical research and practice has been wide-ranging. Many more women doctors and men nurses are practicing today than in the past, and their ways of relating to patients reflect the feminist encouragement of attention to the "whole patient." Women are now routinely included in trials of new drugs and surgical treatments. The gender context of illnesses and disabilities is an intrinsic part of research designs. Women's health is part of medical school curriculums. There has been a proliferation of medical journals devoted to gender-based medicine, women's health and illnesses, and men's health and illnesses.

Our intent in this book is to show how gender, in conjunction with racial and ethnic identification, social class, and sexual orientation, creates different risks and protections for physical illnesses, produces different behavior when ill, elicits different responses in health care personnel, affects the social worth of patients, and influences priorities of treatment, research, and financing. We will concentrate on problems that are located in the body, such as infections, AIDS, or nonfunctioning limbs or senses; and physical processes, such as menstruation and menopause, that in Western society have been transformed into illnesses. These bodily manifestations are often influenced by feelings of stress, anxiety, and depression, but the symptoms or causes are primarily physical. The *context*, however, is *social*, and social contexts are usually gendered—they have different effects on women and men.

Sex Differences and Gender Statuses

Sex and *gender* are often used interchangeably by laypeople and by professionals in science and medicine. In 2001, the U.S. Institute of Medicine issued a book-length report on sex-based differences in human disease (Wizemann and Pardue 2001). In it, reflecting feminist perspectives, the sixteen-member panel of varied professionals struggled to differentiate and define *sex* and *gender*. Their recommendations on terminology were that *sex* should refer "to the reproductive organs and functions that derive from the chromosomal complement," and that *gender* "should be used to refer to a person's self-representation . . . , or how that person is responded to by social institutions on the basis of the individual's gender presentation" (p. 139). The Institute of Medicine's definition of gender implies that people are treated according to how they perceive or present themselves. However, feminist sociologists have demonstrated that people's gender identifications and gender displays are a response to social pressures, which, in turn, are embedded in a gendered social order.

From the social construction perspective, gender is a society's division of people into differentiated categories of "women" and "men." Gender operates at one and the same time as an individual social status, a relational factor, an organizational process, and a system-level social institution. Each level supports and maintains the others, but—and this is the crucial aspect of gender—the effects of gender work top down. When gender is a building block of social orders, it gets built into organizations, floods interactions and relationships, and is a major social identity for individuals.

In the social construction perspective, gender is an intrinsic part of many societies' social orders. Gender divisions are built into the major social organizations of those societies, such as the economy, the family, religion, the arts, and politics. In those societies, gender is a major social status for individuals, with established patterns of expectations and life opportunities. The social construction perspective sees gendering as an ongoing process—with people constantly "doing gender" (West and Zimmerman 1987). Through interaction with caretakers, socialization in childhood, peer pressure in adolescence, and gendered work and family roles, people are divided into two groups and made to be different in behavior, attitudes, and emotions. The content of the differences depends on the society's culture, values, economic and family structure, and past history. The gendered social order produces and maintains these differences. There is a continuous loop-back effect between the gendered social order and the social construction of gender at the organizational, relational, and individual levels. In societies with institutional racism and discrimination by ethnic group and social class, gender is intricately intertwined with these other statuses, forming what Patricia Hill Collins (1990) calls a "matrix of domination." *Gender is therefore multiple: Women and men are not homogenous groupings.*

Bodies and biological differences have also been viewed from a social construction perspective. In this view, gender is not an overlay on biology; rather, biology itself is socially constructed *as* gendered. Sex differences do matter, but the way they matter is a social phenomenon. Menstruation, menopause, pregnancy, and childbirth are biological phenomena that are mediated and experienced socially. Female and male bodies are gendered for femininity and masculinity through sports, exercise, and physical labor. Gendered eating patterns have physiological consequences: Men's rates of coronary heart disease rose precipitously after World War II in Western industrialized countries because they had the privilege of eating more scarce red meat (Lawlor et al. 2001). When a woman moves to a different country, her risk of dying of breast cancer gradually changes, for better or worse, to match the risk in her new place of residence (Kliewer and Smith 1995; Ziegler 1993). As Anne Fausto-Sterling says, "Reading nature is a sociocultural act" (2000, 75).

Sex is also not a simple binary. Sex multiplies into physiological characteristics of children and adults at different stages of the life cycle and by physical abilities. Women's biological states change, depending on whether they are pregnant or not pregnant, between periods or menstruating, pre- or postmenopausal. Men's biological states change with fluctuations in testosterone levels and other hormonal cycles. These within-sex differences must be considered when designing experiments for vaccines, medications, and surgery.

Sex differences occur in a social matrix of gender statuses—gendered patterns of social interaction, gendered expectations for how people should behave in families and workplaces, and gendered social institutions that legally and in informal social practices treat women and men of various racial, ethnic, and social class groups very differently. Medical and biological research has to be both sex-based and gender-based; research designs have to recognize that sex and gender are multiple, not binary, and intertwined in complex ways.

The framework for the gender lens on illness and health is the *transformation of the body through gendered social practices*.[3] These practices start before birth—what a pregnant woman eats, what prenatal technology and care is available to her, what her family and educational and economic status are, what social worth a child of a woman of her racial ethnic group, economic status, and family background is likely to have—all affect the fetus, infant, and growing child as profoundly as genetic inheritance. Social practices produce social bodies all through life and death—and beyond (consider how corpses are handled). Because gender is embedded in the major social institutions of society, such as the economy, the family, politics, and the medical and legal systems, it has a major impact on how the women and men of different social groups are treated in all sectors of life, including health and illness, getting born and dying. Gender is thus one of the most significant factors in the transformation of physical bodies into social bodies. The *gendered body in its social context* is the framework for the analysis of the social construction of illness.

The Social Construction of Illness

Although it is located in the body, illness as a social experience goes far beyond physiology. The process of what comes to be termed a legitimate illness is entrenched in hierarchies of power and economic resources (Brown 1995). Sociologists use the term *medicalization* to explain how life events, including all aspects of the aging process, and social problems such as alcoholism and obesity, come to be defined and managed by health care professionals. Medicalization makes many physiological differences "illnesses" to be treated with examinations, tests, and prescriptions for frequently very expensive drugs. The health care provider is the expert; what the patient knows about his or her own body and his or her own life is not part of prevention, maintenance, or cure.

Medicalization is deeply embedded in financing structures of health care. Making so many physical states into illnesses enhances the capitalist profit motive in countries like the United States. Conversely, it comes into conflict with the cost-cutting practices in countries that have nationalized services. The combination of medicalization and financing structure affects health care professionals' behavior toward patients. If the goal is to increase the patient load, they will be encouraged to call every symptom a treatable illness. If the bottom line is to cut costs, they may neglect rare, time-consuming, or complex medical problems. In all Westernized medical systems, health care providers use the biomedical data produced by research institutions and federal health agencies, whose priorities are shaped by sources of funding. These sources may be pharmaceutical companies, governmental agencies, or private philanthropies. They all have agendas that shape research questions, and they target populations the research is designed to benefit, exploit, or control. Medicalization can thus do too much to make every common symptom an illness treatable by a pill or injection, and too little to prevent illnesses caused by pollution, occupational hazards, poverty, or substance abuse.

For patients, symptoms occur in the context of their lives. These symptoms become an illness through the process of seeking professional help, but the social experience of being a patient also involves kin, colleagues, friends, and one's place in the world. A broken leg may be a simple fracture, but it is experienced entirely differently by a professional athlete, for whom it is a career-stopper, and an office worker, for whom it is an annoying temporary encumbrance. Two illnesses may be easily treated by antibiotics and quite curable, but the social effects of pneumonia are far different from the social consequences of gonorrhea. If you have had gonorrhea, you may want to keep it a secret when you apply for a job. If you have had pneumonia, you may use that as the reason you have to stay home from work with a bad cold.

Because illness is socially constructed, health care providers and patients may see the same set of symptoms (or lack of them) entirely differently. Physicians tend to look first for visible physical symptoms or clear test results. For them, the ideal illness situation is one that produces an unambiguous diagnosis with effective treatment that will cure the disease by removing the symptoms or that will restore the patient to more or less normal functioning. For patients, modified ability to conduct their lives with chronic but treatable conditions is a considerably different situation than a complete cure. A cure restores you to your previous status; a chronic condition forces you to establish new patterns of behavior. Similarly, what the physician may see as unavoidable side effects from necessary treatment, the patient may experience as unwarranted increased pain or discomfort, stress, and financial cost. Patients who feel their doctor has ignored signs of complications or prescribed unnecessary surgery may sue for malpractice. If an HMO defines an illness in a way that deprives a patient of care, the patient may sue for damages. The definition of what constitutes an illness is often an embattled terrain.

The Social Context

The social context is an integral part of any illness. From recognition and attention to symptoms through actions while sick, to coping with recovery or a chronic condition or dying, all of a patient's social characteristics have an effect. This effect is shaped by social networks, work and financial status, family obligations, health care systems, and cultural values. As health care systems change, so does the behavior of patients, caretakers, and health care professionals.

For the greater part of the twentieth century, American medicine was practiced by physicians working alone in their offices, visiting their patients in hospitals, and collecting a fee for their services (Starr 1982). Patients and physicians negotiated with each other directly, but the physician had all the power and prestige. Patients tended to see physicians of their own race and religion, but not their own gender, since women studying medicine were kept to a quota of about 5 to 6 percent in medical schools that admitted them and in hospitals where they did their clinical training (Walsh 1977). One medical school for women survived the professionalization of medicine in the early 1900s—the Women's Medical College of Pennsylvania—but no all-women's hospitals did. Because of religious quotas, Catholic and Jewish men physicians trained in and put their patients into hospitals supported by Catholic and Jewish charities (Solomon 1961). African-American and Hispanic physicians went to federally funded medical schools and used mostly publicly funded hospitals or community-based clinics (Hine 1985; Moldow 1987). Nurses were strictly under physicians' orders (Reverby 1987). Native American and other indigenous healers, although they had many clients in their communities, were not considered legitimate health care workers.

Today, women physicians of all racial ethnic groups make up half or more of most medical school classes in the United States, but medical specialties are not evenly gender-integrated. More nurses and nursing administrators are men. Nurse-practitioners and nurse-midwives are responsible for their own patients. Native and homeopathic health providers, such as acupuncturists and nutritional specialists, are paid for by some health insurance plans.

The major change in the structure of medical care in the United States is the expansion of health maintenance plans (HMOs), where the provider is paid by a third party (insurance agency or the government), the patient's choice of physicians and hospitals is often restricted, and the physician's choice of treatments and medications is confined to what the payer allows. Since the goal of most private health plans is profit, insurers have been extremely influential in creating cost-effective decision models for health care providers. Physicians have lost prestige and authority, but patients have not gained any power in the medical encounter (Freidson 1989). The third party in the negotiation is the payer, a large, for-profit or government bureaucracy that tries to develop one-size-fits-all rules. These include limited hospital stays and ambulatory surgery, where the patient is sent home still needing physical care. Even with visiting health care providers, a family member or friend must be available to be the "nurse" (Glazer 1991). Other important players in Westernized medicine are pharmaceutical companies, which fund many seemingly unbiased clinical trials. Hefty profit margins and expandable markets determine research and development priorities; thus, Viagra for erectile dysfunction gets produced, as well as antidepressants and allergy medications. In such a system, the essence of illness—its diversified social context—is suppressed.

In sum, although all human beings experience the universal physical phenomena of birth, growth, illness, aging, and death, and each individual's experiences of these phenomena are particular, between these universals and these particulars are the similarities that come out of membership in social groups—women and men of various racial categories, ethnicities, and economic classes, living at different times and in different places. Social location produces patterns of health and illness behavior, but equally important in shaping experiences as patients are the actions of professionals encountered in seeking help and the organizational and financial structures of health care systems.

Overview of the Book

This book's focus is a *gender analysis* of the transformation of physiological symptoms into the social reality we call illness. A gender analysis shows how gender is built into almost every aspect of illness in modern society— risks of and protections from different diseases, the perception and response of the patient to symptoms, the organization and delivery of health care, the politics of diagnosis, funding priorities, the problems explored by clinical and scientific researchers, the knowledge and meaning of diseases and their treatment. Each chapter examines a major issue in health and illness through a gender lens perspective. These issues are: *social epidemiology and risks of disease; professional hierarchies and patient-provider interaction; social aspects of physical disability; the politics of diagnosis in premenstrual syndrome and menopause; genital surgeries; and AIDS as a modern plague.* The concluding chapter discusses ways in which the recommendations of *feminist health care* can be applied to all patients.

Chapter 2, "Women Get Sicker, but Men Die Quicker," explains epidemiological rates of death and illness in terms of women's and men's *sociocultural risk factors.* These factors are a combination of gender norms, racial ethnic group membership, economic resources, and social relationships. The social environment and social practices in which risk factors are embedded make different groups of people vulnerable to or protected from the causes of illness. Social epidemiological statistics are influenced by methodological issues, such as what questions are asked and how the answers are categorized, as well as by the reliability of techniques of information-gathering and measurement. Unless women and men of different racial groups and social classes are included in a sample, researchers have no way of making socially useful comparisons of health status, health practices, and risk-taking behavior. These statistics are usually not value-free; priorities are set by those who have the power and resources to get answers to the questions of importance to them. You might say that what counts gets counted.

Chapter 3, "Hierarchies in Health Care," analyzes *gendered and professional power differences* and the interactive behavior of health care providers and patients. Whether the physician is a woman or a man influences how much attention is paid to women's and men's presenting complaints, especially what kind of tests are ordered and what kind of treatment is recommended. Nurse-practitioners are trained to look for the interaction of psychosocial factors with physiological symptoms and treat them simultaneously. Similarities and differences in culture and lifestyle also influence the interpretation of symptoms.

Chapter 4, "Gender and Disability," examines the *gendered contradictions and status dilemmas* of people with disabilities. It defines disability as a permanent social status that is only partly shaped by medical encounters. More influential is the availability of technological and environmental supports that allow people with disabilities to hold jobs and create families. Both women and men have benefited from the successes of the disability rights movement, but the special needs of women with disabilities for jobs, sexual relationships, and a family life have not been so squarely faced. The gendered expectations of women and men create constraints for both, but women with disabilities have fewer opportunities for long-term relationships. They need unbiased professional services, especially around sexuality and procreation. Another gender difference that impacts on those with disabilities is the expectation that caregivers will be women. Thus, if people with disabilities have special needs to enable them to live mainstream lives, then women with disabilities have even more specialized needs.

Chapter 5, "If a Situation Is Defined as Real . . .," examines the ways in which *premenstrual tension and menopausal mood swings* are socially and medically constructed. Symptoms individually experienced at different points in women's procreative life cycle are medicalized into physiological and psychological syndromes. Some women may pay little attention to premenstrual tension, menstrual cramps, and menopausal hot flashes, while others may need treatment for them. But if these occurrences are routinely labeled illnesses, then all women will be considered "sick" or not able to function normally. The part that medicine as a social institution plays in legitimizing appropriate behavior in women can be seen as a form of social control.

Chapter 6, "Genital Surgeries," looks at the *gender and cultural conflicts* in ritual and medical genital surgery. Although the social contexts of female and male ritual genital surgery, surgery on intersex children, and routine medical circumcisions are very different, the issues are similar—adults make decisions about genital surgery on infants and children in the name of cultural conformity. In ritual genital surgery, adults surgically modify a child's body to make the child appropriately feminine or masculine. The same goal governs genital surgery on children born with ambiguous-looking external genitalia. The body undergoes a profound social as well as physical transformation, a transformation that is, above all, gendered.

The debates over genital surgeries are confounded by opposing cultural, religious, and medical perspectives. Cultural traditions clash with human rights issues; religious beliefs clash with parental reluctance to do bodily harm to their children. Medical researchers argue over the risks and benefits of what seems like minor surgery. Gender weaves into all of these debates because they all involve beliefs about male and female sexuality, how female and male bodies should look, and how to prevent sexually transmitted diseases from spreading.

Chapter 7, "A Modern Plague," takes illness into the moral realm of social identities contaminated by *stigmatized diseases*. AIDS (acquired immunodeficiency syndrome) is an epidemic imbued with gender, sexuality, class, and racial ethnic discrimination. AIDS is very much affected by gender in its transmission and treatment. Its physical ravages and social costs today fall most heavily on poor women and men who live in developing countries. The discourse and dynamics around AIDS is a prime example of how sickness is reflective of cultural views of women and men, homosexuals and heterosexuals, poor and rich, people of color and Whites, "foreigners" and "natives."

How HIV-positive status and the symptoms of AIDS are reacted to and treated reflects heterosexual, bisexual, and homosexual relationships; the constellation of patient, practitioners, and lay caretakers; community attitudes; cultural values; and the politics of medical bureaucracies and government agencies. Those who are known to be HIV-positive or to show the signs of full-blown AIDS have been stigmatized for their sexual practices or drug use and out of fear of contagion from their semen, blood, or breast milk. From negotiations over condom use between sexual partners to allocation of funds for research and treatment by national and international agencies, AIDS literally and figuratively embodies the material, experiential, and symbolic gendered construction of illness.

Chapter 8, "Healing Social Bodies in Social Worlds," looks at the conflict between the ways in which professionals and laypeople define medical reality and proposes an alternative—*feminist health care*. Such care sees the patient and the health care professional as equals in the medical encounter. The professional knows more about illnesses and their treatment in general, but the patient knows more about her or his particular case. Feminist health care advocates recommend that before professionals apply general medical science, they should understand the patient's social and environmental contexts and the patient's history with the particular disease. When professionals prescribe a course of treatment, they should tell the patient not only what the risks and side effects are, but also advise as to the advantages and disadvantages of other courses of treatment and nontreatment. Then the patient should decide what he or she wants to do, and expect the continued support and help of the professional, even if the professional's first choice for treatment was rejected.

Feminist health care is for all people—men as well as women, children as well as adults. Feminist health care encompasses major transformations of the existing structures of funding, training, and providing biomedical health care. Feminist perspectives on health and illness have been incorporated into medical and nursing schools' curricula, but they need to be reinforced in clinical training and built into day-to-day practices by organizational policies that encourage enough time for listening to patients and pay for diverse types of treatment. These are idealistic goals, but when shared by both providers and consumers of care, they empower many who might otherwise find it difficult to confront the limitations of current biomedical health care systems.

Notes

1. See Freidson 1970a, 1970b; Mishler 1981, 1984; Waitzkin 1983, 1991.

2. For overall feminist critiques, see Fisher 1986; Martin 1992; Todd 1989; Ruzek 1978.

3. For theories of the social body, see Featherstone et al. 1991; Shilling 1993; Turner 1984, 1992.

CHAPTER 2

Women Get Sicker, but Men Die Quicker:
Social Epidemiology

In any gender-dichotomized society, the fact that we are born biologically female or male means that our environments will be different: we will live different lives. Because our biology and how we live are dialectically related and build on one another, we cannot vary gender and hold the environment constant. (Hubbard 1990: 128)

There is a saying in epidemiology—"women get sicker, but men die quicker." It is a succinct way of summing up the illness and death rates of women and men in modern industrialized societies. These rates are the cumulative effects of social, environmental, and physical processes and of individual, community, and society-wide behaviors. To a very great extent, they reflect the gender system and the effects of differential life experiences of racial ethnic groups.

Social epidemiology studies disease and death rates from a perspective that emphasizes "the social distribution and social determinants of states of health" (Berkman and Kawachi 2000). The social epidemiologist's task is to explain variances in *morbidity* (rates of illness) and *mortality* (rates of death) and to tease out the causes of persistent group differences. The most familiar rates are those for life expectancy, which are a kind of summary of the physical, environmental, and social conditions that affect how long a newborn can expect to live.

In industrialized countries, in the early years of the twentieth century, women started to outlive men by several years. In the new century, in the same countries, women can outlive men by almost ten years.[1] There are two perspectives used to explain the virtually global trend of higher life expectancy rates for women in industrialized countries. One perspective relies on a biological argument about the protective effects of estrogen and the potentially toxic effects of testosterone (Perls and Fretts 1998). However, this perspective does not attend to historical changes in life expectancies nor does it take into account racial ethnic and social class differences. A more complex argument claims that life expectancies are the result of a combination of social and biological factors.

Women have not always lived so much longer than men. In Europe and North America, the gendered gap in life expectancy grew as economic development and social change encouraged greater control over the size of families and wider application of innovative public health measures. Death in childbirth, a large contributor to women's life expectancy rates, decreased with the rise of modern medicine. Simultaneously, the gendered division of labor has exposed men to greater occupational risks. In many industrialized countries, as family income increases, men eat more meat and fatty foods than women do, and have higher rates of coronary heart disease. Compared to men in the nineteenth century, men today smoke more and exercise less.

Men and women have different risks and protections throughout their lifetimes—male fetuses and newborns, for example, are more fragile physically and die at a higher rate than females. Men and women have different social risks as well—women from dying in childbirth and from domestic violence, men from getting killed in war and in street fighting. Men are more likely to engage in risky health-related behaviors, such as smoking, drug abuse, and dangerous sexual activities, which make them more vulnerable to heart disease, strokes, and sexually transmitted disorders. All of these factors add up to different life expectancies.

The pattern of longer life expectancy for men and women as a country modernizes, as well as the gender gap favoring women by several years, is not a constant. Russia and other eastern European countries have seen reduced life expectancies for women and men, and it currently has the largest gender disparity among industrialized countries, 66.4 years for female babies but just 56.1 years for males.[2] Researchers cite the high incidence of men's alcohol abuse, which leads to high rates of accidents, violence, and cardiovascular disease (McKee and Shkolnikov 2001). Gender differences are minimized when women and men live and work in similar unpressured environments. A comparison of the health status of 230 women and men on two Israeli kibbutzim, where work and family life are communal and health care is free, found that they were alike in their health status and illness behavior and that the men had life expectancies as long as those of the women (Anson et al. 1990).

In the United States, racial differences increase the gender gap in life expectancy. Life expectancy for a White infant born in the late 1990s is five and a half years longer for a girl than for a boy, but for Black infants, the difference is seven years. The combined racial and sex difference between the longest life expectancy (White women) and the shortest (Black men) is over twelve years (see table 2.1). Black women and men not only die earlier, but are prone to more illnesses, physical traumas, and missed or incorrect diagnoses throughout their lives than White women and men. Paradoxically, although White women have the longest life expectancy, they have more reported illnesses throughout their adult lives than White men. Although women as well as men are subject to heart diseases, cancers, and other life-threatening physical problems, on the whole, women live longer than men in industrialized countries because men get these killer diseases earlier (Verbrugge 1989).

Table 2.1

United States Life Expectancy, by Gender and White and Black Racial Categories

	ALL			WHITE			BLACK		
Year		Men	Women		Men	Women		Men	Women
1998	76.7	73.8	79.5	77.3	74.5	80.0	71.3	67.6	74.8

Source: "Death and Death Rates by Race and Sex." National Vital Health Statistics Reports. 2000. CDC Web page.

In contrast, in societies where women's social status is very low, their life expectancy is reduced by a combination of social factors—eating last and eating less, complications of frequent childbearing and sexually transmitted diseases because they have no power to demand abstinence or condom use, infections and hemorrhages following childbirth, neglect of symptoms of illness until severe, and restricted access to modern health care (Santow 1995; see table 2.2). The relationship between women's health

Table 2.2

Global Life Expectancies, By Ranks and Gender
(SELECTED COUNTRIES)

COUNTRY	RANK	OVERALL	MEN	WOMEN
Japan	1	74.5	71.9	77.2
Australia	2	73.2	70.8	75.5
France	3	73.1	69.3	76.9
Sweden	4	73.0	71.2	74.9
Spain	5	72.8	69.8	75.7
Italy	6	72.7	70.0	75.4
Greece	7	72.5	70.5	74.6
Switzerland	8	72.5	69.5	75.5
Canada	12	72.0	70.0	74.0
Netherlands	13	72.0	69.6	74.4
United Kingdom	14	71.7	69.7	73.7
Norway	15	71.7	68.8	74.6
Belgium	16	71.6	68.7	74.6
Germany	22	70.4	67.4	73.5
Israel	23	70.4	69.2	71.6
United States	24	70.0	67.5	72.6
China	81	62.3	61.2	63.3
Russia	91	61.3	56.1	66.4
Brazil	111	59.1	55.2	62.9
Philippines	113	58.9	57.1	60.7
Egypt	115	58.5	58.6	58.3
Pakistan	124	55.9	55.0	56.8
India	134	53.2	52.8	53.5
Korea	137	52.3	51.4	53.1
Bangladesh	140	49.9	50.1	49.8
Haiti	153	43.8	42.4	45.2
South Africa	160	39.8	38.6	41.0
Niger	190	29.1	28.1	30.1
Sierra Leone	191	25.9	25.8	26.0

Source: "WHO Issues New Healthy Life Expectancy Rankings: Japan Number One in New 'Healthy Life' System." 2000. World Health Organization (WHO) Web site. These life expectancies were calculated using the WHO's Disability Adjusted Life Expectancy (DALE) measure. As WHO states, the DALE "summarizes the expected number of years to be lived in what might be termed the equivalent of 'full health.' To calculate DALE, the years of ill-health are weighted according to severity and subtracted from the expected overall life expectancy to give the equivalent years of healthy life."

and their social status is starkly demonstrated by how care is allocated within the family in many traditional societies:

> A lower-status individual, such as a young female, was likely to be treated only with home remedies; when assistance was sought outside the household it was more likely to be from a traditional than a modern therapist. A higher-status individual, such as a male of almost any age or an adult mother of sons, was likely to be taken directly to a private medical practitioner. (Santow 1995, 154)

When the causes of disease are genetic and physiological, environmental exposure often determines their onset, and social resources influence their outcome. For example, sickle cell anemia and breast cancer cluster in different racial ethnic groups, but access to knowledge, healthy environments, and up-to-date treatment cluster by social class. "The reason is that resources like knowledge, money, power, prestige, and social connectedness are transportable from one situation to another, and as health-related situations change, those who command the most resources are best able to avoid risks, diseases, and consequences of disease" (Link and Phelan 1995, 87). Morbidity and mortality rates are therefore useful for policy recommendations only when accompanied by data on social factors, such as economic resources, access to health services, community supports, and cultural values. What Nancy Krieger calls "ecosocial theory" asks "how we literally incorporate, biologically, social relations (such as those of social class, race/ethnicity, and gender) into our bodies, thereby focusing on who and what drives population patterns of health, disease, and well being" (1996, 135).

Social epidemiologists, health care providers, policy makers, and the media use morbidity and mortality rates to assess the health of groups of people and to distribute social resources. And, just like health and illness, the reliability of these epidemiological rates is also influenced by social factors. Most importantly, rates vary depending on how the epidemiological data has been collected and analyzed. For example, reports of sudden infant death syndrome (SIDS), defined as the sudden death of an infant less than a year old that cannot be explained by any other factors, are more common where mothers are poor, have little education, and are from non-White racial ethnic groups. Biological or medical models predict a random distribution over social groups. The high rates for children from non-White racial ethnic groups may be the result of overreporting—attributing unexplained deaths to SIDS when the families are poor more often than when they are rich (Nam et al. 1989).

In addition to over- and underreporting, another measurement problem in social epidemiology is how illness is assessed: Is it by days off from work, visits to health care professionals, days in hospital, medication use, or self-assessment? Women are more likely than men to take days off, see health care professionals, use medication, and assess themselves as sicker. That is, women are more likely to attend to symptoms than men are for a variety of reasons, among them familiarity with the health care system through gynecological checkups, pregnancies, and taking children to pediatricians. Men are encouraged from childhood to be stoical, and so are not as likely to see a doctor for nonserious health problems. When they do get sick, they are more likely to be hospitalized and less likely to get psychosocial support (Moynihan 1998). Thus, by epidemiological measures, women are sicker than men most of their adult lives, but the health-seeking behavior that produces their high illness rates probably increases their longevity. Women are not more fragile physically than men, just more self-protective of their health.

Still another social epidemiological issue is immediate and long-term causes of death. In establishing causal models of death and disease, epidemiologists try to find a single cause-and-effect relationship. However, they must contend with multiple social variables that affect an individual's health. For an eighty-five-year-old woman, pneumonia is often the official cause of death, but long-term causes may be just as significant. These might be poor nutrition, run-down housing, and no support services. But in our biomedical world, poverty is never an official cause of death.

The statistical patterns of morbidity and mortality—who gets sick with what and who dies when from what—are outcomes of individual behavior shaped by cultural and social factors, such as availability of clean water and good food, access to health care, medical knowledge and technology, and protection from environmental pollution, occupational traumas, and social hazards like war, violent crime, rape, and battering. For the individual, health is as much affected by combined social statuses (gender, racial ethnic group, social class, occupation, and place of residence) as by personal choices. Indeed, individual behavior is heavily circumscribed by social statuses—not everyone chooses health risks; for some people, health risks are built into their daily lives (Haynes et al. 2000). On a broader social system level, rates of illness and death are significantly affected by the behavior of health care providers, the policies of health care institutions and agencies, and the financial support of state and national governments for research and treatment.

According to Robert Staples,

> Black men suffer a disproportionate burden of illness. The drug and alcoholism rate for blacks, for example, is about four times higher than whites. Whereas black men suffer higher rates of diabetes, strokes and a variety of chronic illnesses, they are also at the mercy of public hospitals, and, therefore, are the first victims of government cutbacks. When they do go to a hospital, they are more likely to receive inadequate treatment. (1995, 123; also see Smedley et al. 2002)

Because social factors are so intertwined, gender cannot be easily separated out. To give you an idea of some of the gendered patterns of morbidity and mortality that are the combined result of risky and protective behavior, environments, social expectations, and economic and other resources, we present a gender analysis of health behaviors through the life cycle—birth, adolescence and young adulthood, adulthood, old age, and death.

Birthing and Getting Born: Have Money or Be a Boy

For pregnant women, economic resources can spell the difference between life and death. For their infants, in poor countries that favor men, all the advantages go to boys. The physical hazards that produce infertility are evenly incurred by men and women, but the social stigma and biomedical treatments are much more difficult for women.

Childbirth and Infancy

One of the important contributors to women's longer life expectancy in the twentieth century is the reduction of illness and death in childbirth.[3] The use of antibiotics for puerperal infections ("childbed fevers") and surgical interventions to prevent heavy blood loss have made dying in childbirth a rare occurrence in many countries. However, because of uneven access to prenatal care and safe abortions and inadequate treatment of childbirth complications, women in the child-bearing years still suffer from high mortality and morbidity rates in many parts of the world (Dixon-Mueller 1994; Sundari 1994). A critical public health issue, maternal mortality rates are acutely different between developed and developing nations (98 percent of all maternal deaths occur in developing countries). As the World Health Organization reports, in some countries, over the course of her child-bearing years, one woman in ten dies from a pregnancy-related cause. In contrast, in the most industrialized countries, including the United States, the chances of dying in childbirth average around one in 4,000.[4] In addition, the health of the mother directly affects the health of the infant. In industrialized countries, "the condition that enables us to predict with the greatest accuracy whether or not a baby will be stillborn, sick, malformed, premature, or will die in the first year of life, is the mother's socioeconomic status. If she belongs to a disadvantaged social class this means, among other things, low income, poor health, hard domestic and extra-domestic work, low educational level, and bad housing" (Romito and Hovelaque 1987, 254).

The more economic resources a country has and the more equally distributed they are, the better the health status and the lower the death rate of women in childbirth and their newborns in their first year. Physiologically, girl babies are stronger at birth, and the female hormones generated at puberty are protective until menopause. However, women's longer life expectancy in developed countries, compared to men, reflects the effects of a healthier environment, better health care, and good nutrition, which are indicative of enough economic resources to feed women and girls as well as men and boys and to give pregnant women good health care (see table 2.3). Another set of statistics related to female life expectancy is literacy rates and family size. Educated women contribute income to families

Table 2.3

Estimates of Maternal Mortality, by United Nations Regions (1995)

REGION	MATERNAL DEATHS PER 100,000 LIVE BIRTHS	ANNUAL NUMBER OF MATERNAL DEATHS	LIFETIME RISK OF MATERNAL DEATH— 1 IN:
WORLD TOTAL	400	515,000	75
MORE DEVELOPED REGIONS	21	2,800	2,500
LESS DEVELOPED REGIONS	440	512,000	60
LEAST DEVELOPED COUNTRIES	1,000	230,000	16

Source: "UN Agencies Issue Joint Statement for Reducing Maternal Mortality." 1999. WHO Web site.

and leave the home to work in the public sphere; they have fewer and more widely spaced pregnancies and their maternal mortality rates drop.

In countries that put a high premium on having sons, neglect and infanticide of baby girls by poorer families and deliberate abortions of female fetuses after prenatal sex testing by wealthier couples has resulted in an imbalanced sex ratio (proportion of boys to girls or men to women) (Renteln 1992). Africa, Europe, and North America have a sex ratio of 95 girls to 100 boys, considered balanced because more boys than girls are born to compensate for the higher natural death rate of male children. In China, India, Bangladesh, and West Asia, the sex ratio in the 1990s has been 94 girls to 100 boys, and in Pakistan, 90 girls to 100 boys. Given the number of men, there should have been about 30 million more women in India, and 38 million more women in China (Coale and Banister 1994).

These numbers do not necessarily reflect a complete devaluation of girls but rather a preference for boys if family size has to be limited. In China, for example, peasants feel that the ideal family is a son and a daughter; a daughter is an emotional and financial backup in case the son proves unfilial in the parents' old age (Greenhalgh and Li 1995). State policy, however, has forcefully discouraged a second child if the first is a son and forbidden a third child in almost all cases. Thus, many families have one or two sons and no daughters.

In India, the official state ideology of fertility control has been small families in which daughters and sons are equally valued. The official image of the modern Indian woman is a mother whose priorities are the welfare of her family, and, by limiting the number of children, the welfare of the nation. Women's burden of responsible parenthood is not matched by sexual or social autonomy or a diminished cultural preference for sons. From the point of view of Indian feminists, it is not surprising, therefore, that resistance to contraception and clandestine female infanticide and abortions of female fetuses persist (Chatterjee and Riley 2001).[5]

If countries have state programs to reduce or to increase their birthrates, women's wishes are foregone in the interests of official population policies. The rhetoric of women's liberation or women's empowerment as honored mothers may be invoked to gain women's support for having fewer or more children, but it is the interests of the state, not women, that prevail in "the freighted politics flowing from the knotting of woman/nation/population" (Greenhalgh 2001, 851). Even ostensibly "hands-off" societies subtly or openly influence procreative decisions (Meyers 2001).

Infertility

Infertility is medically defined as no pregnancy after a year of trying. It has been more detrimental physiologically and socially for women than for men, even though male infertility seems to be on the rise and is very difficult to treat.[6]

In men, chemotherapy, ulcer and high blood pressure medications, alcohol, marijuana, and anabolic steroids for bulking up muscles can all lower sperm counts. In the last decade, research from sixty-one studies implicates a global environment riddled with toxic pollutants in significantly lowering sperm counts throughout the world (Swan and Elkin 1999).

In both women and men, there is little protection against workplace exposure to fertility-reducing toxins. Nurses and anesthetists are exposed to radiation and powerful anesthetics, and assemblers in electronics factories work with potentially harmful solvents (Draper 1993). In 1991, the U.S. Supreme Court decided that employers could not use protection of the fetus as a rationale for barring fertile women from hazardous jobs. The decision to take a job that might cause infertility is now up to workers themselves (including men at risk of sperm deformity). The government could insist that employers reduce all workers' exposure to occupational hazards or equip them with protective devices.[7] In addition to job-related hazards, sexually transmitted diseases, malnutrition, and inadequate health care have contributed to higher rates of infertility among African Americans, and they are less likely to have access to expensive procreative technologies (Nsiah-Jefferson and Hall 1989). For all groups, a significant cause of infertility in later life are teenage *chlamydia* infections, a very common bacterial sexually transmitted disease that may have no symptoms and therefore go undetected and untreated (Walsh et al. 2000). In addition, participation in the public sector and the effectiveness of contraceptive devices have led many women to decide to begin families later in life, when fertility may have diminished. In the United States from 1975 to 1997, there has been a steady increase of thirty- to thirty-four-year-old women's first birth rate (Ventura et al. 2000).

Because so much of the treatment for infertility takes place inside women's bodies, women have more at stake but less bargaining power in the decisions over what to do about not being able to conceive. Whether the woman or the man is infertile, the woman is usually the one who initially seeks help. If she is determined to have a biological child with her male partner, she has to assure his willingness to undergo demands like intercourse at ovulation and masturbation to produce fresh sperm. She will also need sympathy and emotional support throughout the days, months, and often years of repeated attempts to get pregnant. Conversely, if she refuses to undergo fertility treatments, her infertile male partner's opportunity to have a biological child in this relationship is lost. This imbalance in the demands of treatment sets up the dynamics of gender bargaining in male infertility (Lorber 1989; Lorber and Bandlamudi 1993).

There are several assisted reproductive technologies readily available in many countries. They may or may not be covered under insurance plans or national health services, and some (such as surrogacy) are illegal in some countries. Table 2.4 describes these procedures and, where available, their success rates.

Willingness to undergo repeated infertility treatments, even if they are unsuccessful, may be a rational decision for women, since families, the media, and the medical system all favor undergoing treatment (Koch 1990). By going through them, a woman proves to herself, her mate, and her family members that she has done everything she could to have a biological child with her male partner. Donor eggs and sperm and embryo adoption have also made it feasible for single women, women with women partners, and older women to have children that are biologically their "own."[8] Not being able to conceive does not harm physically, but socially and psychologically; the treatments, however, can be physically as well as emotionally and financially costly, especially for women.

Adolescence and Young Adulthood: Good and Bad Social Pressures

Teenagers and young adults face particular risks that threaten their well-being, risks that are socially produced by their environments and by peer pressures, such as pregnancies and eating disorders. The lives of poor young men of color are the most endangered of all groups in the United States, exposing them to a host of physical and emotional traumas.

Teenage Pregnancy

Pregnancy soon after menarche is considered the norm in all but highly industrialized societies, where teenage childbearing is considered a social and political problem. From a health perspective, there are detrimental effects of pregnancy on the body of a growing girl and dangers of prematurity and low birth weight in their babies. From a social perspective, there are

Table 2.4

Assisted Reproductive Technologies (ART), with Success Rates

Technology	Description	Success Rate
Donor Insemination (DI, formerly known as artificial insemination)	Semen from either an unknown donor through a semen bank or from a male friend or relative is inserted either into the vagina (Intra Cervical Insemination) or directly into the cervix (Intra Uterine Insemination). Fresh or frozen semen can be used.	IUI pregnancy rate is 12.4 percent per cycle.[a]
Oocyte Donation (also known as egg donation)	Female donors are given drugs to stimulate the production of eggs. These eggs are harvested at ovulation and inseminated with male partner's or donor sperm. When they develop into embryos, they are implanted into the adopter's womb. Oocyte donation is typically used by women who have premature ovarian failure (under 40 years of age) or who are perimenopausal (over 40 years of age and 5-10 years before menopause).	Pregnancy rates vary depending upon the recipient's age.
In Vitro Fertilization (IVF)	Hormones are administered to increase production of ova. They are removed and fertilized with sperm in a petri dish. Gametes are incubated for a day or two until the resultant cell division produces an embryo that can be implanted into the woman's womb.[b]	24.9 percent live birth rate, according to the 1998 CDC's survey of 360 ART clinics in the United States.[c]
Intracyto-plasmic Sperm Injection (ICSI)	A single active sperm cell is injected directly into a previously surgically removed oocyte. The resultant embryo is implanted into a woman's body. ICSI allows previously subfertile or infertile men to participate in reproduction with their biological gametes.	Clinical pregnancy rate is between 31.6 percent and 36.8 percent.[d]
Embryo Adoption	A previously created embryo is implanted and gestated in the womb of a woman who did not provide the ovum. The gestational mother is designated as the biological mother. If adopted by a heterosexual couple, the designated father is usually not the sperm donor.	N/A
Surrogacy	A woman carries the fetus for another woman. The fetus may or may not be biologically related to a member of the adoptive family. ART may or may not be used to impregnate the gestational carrier.	N/A

[a]Hendin et al., 2000.
[b]Fredericks, Paulson and DeCherney, 1987.
[c]"Assisted Reproductive Technology Success Rates." National Summary and Fertility Clinics Reports, 1998 and 2000. CDC Web site.
[d]Cayan et al., 2001.

the questions of why teenage boys and girls want to have babies and what happens to those girls who do get pregnant. The major social problem for the teenage mother is the risk of ending up in poverty if she is not already poor or staying poor if she is.

Statistics of teenage pregnancy in the United States by racial and ethnic group show rates for Black and Hispanic teens to be twice as high as those for White teens; these differences are attributed to multiple factors, including contraceptive use, age of first intercourse, and amount of sexual activity thereafter (Ventura et al. 2000). In the last decade, there has been a continued decline in the teen birth rate in the United States, with a 21.4 percent drop from 1990 to 1998 among 15- to 17-year-olds.[9] The largest decline was among Black teens in the same age group—32.1 percent—and the smallest among Hispanic teens—11.8 percent. Hispanic cultures are sometimes contradictory about nonmarital pregnancies, condemning sexuality outside of marriage but valuing children. The positive attitudes towards fatherhood among young men in many cultures, and their intentions to play a significant role in the lives of their children and their children's mothers, also make it difficult for teenage girls to practice birth control or have an abortion (Anderson 1989; Marsiglio 1988).

Changing social trends, such as more effective contraceptive use by sexually experienced teenagers, are reflected in the recent decline in teenage pregnancies in the United States. Participation in high school athletics is protective against teen pregnancy for girls (Sabo et al. 1999). Thanks to changing views of athletic femininity and equalization of funding for girls' sports, girls are increasingly seeking self-esteem in these arenas (Dworkin and Messner 1999).[10] In general, the incidence of teenage pregnancy is low where sex education is part of the school curriculum and contraceptives and early abortions are widely available (Jones and Forrest 1985).

Endangered Species

Even when young women become pregnant, they are less vulnerable to early mortality than the young men of their racial ethnic groups. Because of multiple risk factors, young African-American men living in disadvantaged environments are the most likely to die before they reach adulthood. In 1998, in the United States, the leading cause of death for all individuals in the 5- to 44-year-old age range is accidents, largely motor vehicle.[11] However, the leading cause of death for young Black men aged 15 to 24 in 1998 was homicide. Because of the 1990s trend of early death rates due to homicides, suicides, and accidents, young African-American men have been called an endangered species (Gibbs 1988; Staples 1995).

Criminalization of Black men has led to overrepresentation in the prison system; they comprised 45.7 percent of the incarcerated in the United States in 1999. There are significant health concerns for men in prisons, including injury, rape, AIDS/HIV, tuberculosis, hepatitis, and mental illness. Although it is well known that rape is common in prisons, it is difficult for the social epidemiologist to calculate rates. Prisoners' rights are generally not deemed important or necessary, as evidenced by the fact that nearly half the states do not collect statistics on rape in prisons. Lack of prevention tactics for rape and drug addiction and lack of treatment for latent infections have created a health crisis for men in prison, with AIDS and hepatitis rates much higher for men in prisons than in comparable groups who are not incarcerated (Kantor 1998; Rhode 2001).

Young men's "taste for risk" has been attributed to sociobiological factors (Wilson and Daly 1985), but more plausible explanations are the seductiveness of danger, displays of heterosexuality and masculinity, and, for Black men, despair over the future (Staples 1995). African-American men who have sex with men are less likely to identify as gay or disclose they are gay. This social stigma increases the difficulty of reaching these men with AIDS prevention and treatment (Kennamer et al. 2000). Although there is a high incidence of HIV infection and AIDS in young Black and Hispanic men, especially when they are intravenous drug users, the consequent AIDS-related illnesses and deaths occur later on, between the ages of 29 and 41 (Kranczer 1995). Another risk factor is the recruitment into often violent sports, which can be a path to higher education for poor and working-class boys (Messner 1992). The few who go on to become successful professional athletes have only a few years to make it, and they cannot afford to be sidelined by injuries. "Playing hurt" and repeated orthopedic surgeries have a high physical toll. Injuries, alcoholism, drug abuse, obesity, and heart disease take about fifteen years off the life expectancy of professional football players in the United States (Messner 1992, 71).

Making the Body Beautiful

Anorexia (self-starvation) and *bulimia* (binge eating and induced vomiting) are extreme ways to lose weight in order to meet Western cultural standards of beauty and to maintain control over one's body (Bordo 1993; Brumberg 1997; Gremillion 2002). Eating disorders are extremely difficult to reverse and can lead to hospitalizations and even death (Ben-Tovim et al. 2001).

Otherwise well protected against health risks, young White middle-class college women who are dissatisfied with their body image are vulnerable to eating disorders (Cooley and Toray 2001).[12] Different cultures think thinness or heftiness is beautiful in women (Miller and Pumariega 2001). The significance of society's views of compulsory heterosexuality and femininity are highlighted by research comparing heterosexual women, who are subject to pressure from the media and the significant men in their lives to stay thin to be sexually attractive, and lesbians, whose views of beauty are not influenced by men's opinions. Lesbians are heavier than comparable heterosexual women, more satisfied with their bodies, and less likely to have eating disorders (Herzog et al. 1992).

Women and men college athletes are prone to anorexia and bulimia when they have to diet to stay in a weight class (Andersen 1990; Black 1991). A study of 695 athletes in 15 college sports found that 1.6 percent of the men and 4.2 percent of the women met the American Psychiatric Association's criteria for anorexia, and 14.2 percent of the men and 39.2 percent of the women met the criteria for bulimia (Burckes-Miller and Black 1991). The reasons for strict weight control are not standards of beauty but the pressures of competition, to meet weight category requirements, to increase speed and height, and to be able to be lifted and carried easily in performances. Eating disorders here are an occupational risk taken not only by young athletes but by dancers, models, jockeys, and fitness instructors, as well as professional gymnasts, figure skaters, runners, swimmers, and wrestlers.

Men and boys also have idealized body images fueled by exposure to childhood toys, like superheros and action figures, and the athletic entertainment industry, such as the World Wrestling Federation (Pope et al. 2000). Attaining this ideal masculine physique may lead to unhealthy practices. In the United States, since 1991, the use and abuse of anabolic steroids, synthetic substances that promote growth of skeletal muscles, has increased annually for tenth graders.[13] Team doctors routinely inject painkillers and cortisone so injured players can play with injuries, and they supply amphetamines to enhance performance and steroids to increase muscle mass.

Steroid use among women and men body builders who enter competitions is endemic, despite their virilizing effects in women and feminizing effects in men (Fussell 1993; Mansfield and McGinn 1993). Some of the physical side effects of steroid abuse include baldness, impotence and sterility, heart disease, and liver and kidney damage.

Adulthood: Health by Choice or by Circumstances?

Many of the risky health behaviors in adulthood, such as drinking and smoking cigarettes, seem to be a matter of individual choice. But a closer look reveals that social factors linked to gender, racial ethnic group, and economic class produce the situational circumstances that influence health-related behaviors.

A study of 4,099 White women and men and 888 Black women and men living in New York State found that Black women were most likely to abstain from drinking (Barr et al. 1993). Black men in this study were more likely than White men to abstain, but also most likely, of all four groups, to be heavy drinkers when they did drink. A study of gendered styles of drinking showed that women of all racial ethnic groups who drank were less likely than men to become visibly intoxicated and to abandon control, behavior that would be considered unfeminine (Robbins and Martin 1993). When economic status was added to the analysis, it was found that the poorest and least educated Black men had significantly higher rates of alcohol and illicit drug consumption and alcohol-related problems, such as accidents and run-ins with the police, boss, fellow workers, and family members. They are, as a result, more likely to suffer from high blood pressure and die early of coronary artery disease, especially if they also smoke (Staples 1995).

There are significant differences in the use of legal and illegal drugs among women and men. From 1992 to 1997, regular cocaine use increased for women but men's cocaine use declined slightly.[14] There is also a high incidence of reports of abuse in childhood, domestic violence, and substance abuse among women who seek treatment for alcohol and other drug problems.[15] When women do seek treatment for drug addiction, they often face discouraging obstacles. Many clinics do not provide child care and many residential treatment programs do not admit women with children (Breitbart et al. 1994).

Women are more than twice as likely as men to be prescribed tranquilizers and sleeping pills, but men often obtain such medications from women—their wives, sisters, or friends—when they are under stress (Ettorre and Riska 1995). Both women and men physicians prescribe these medications to women more than they do to men with similar difficulties, but men physicians are significantly more likely to do so (Taggart et al. 1993). Addiction to these legally prescribed drugs is also a more serious problem for women than for men (Pincus et al. 1998). Elizabeth Ettorre and Elianne Riska (1995) argue that both the gendered use patterns and the prescribing patterns reflect powerlessness: Prescribing tranquilizers for women stressed out by their triple duties as wives, mothers, and paid workers treats the symptoms, not the causes, which women physicians are more likely to recognize. When men in difficult social situations ask sympathetic women they know rather than their men physicians for tranquilizers, the same gender dynamics of status seem to be at issue.

Homicide rates are greater for disadvantaged men but, paradoxically, higher for educated women in the labor force. A cross-national, longitudinal comparison of eighteen industrialized countries found that as women's lives between 1950 and 1985 moved away from traditional roles, they were more likely to be murdered (Gartner 1990). The authors argue that although women confined to the home are subject to violence from husbands and other men relatives, women who work for pay, especially in nontraditional occupations, and single women living on their own are also vulnerable to being killed by acquaintances and strangers.

Work and Family: Protection and Danger

Jobs and families are complex variables with good and bad effects on the physical and mental health of women and men. Both are arenas for social support, which is beneficial to health; both are sometimes hazardous environments with detrimental physical and emotional effects (Chavkin 1984).

Work-Family Demands and Rewards

Although having a paid job outside the home usually enhances women's physical and mental health, jobs can be physically hazardous to women as well as men. Homicide is the leading cause of injury and death for working women (it ranks second for men), with 163 women murdered at work in 1998.[16] Many women's jobs are as physically dangerous as some men's jobs (Messing 1997). For example, hospitals expose nurses to infections, radiation, and dangerous chemicals. The home can be a dangerous work environment, too, full of toxic chemicals and potential allergens.

The job and the home can each produce high levels of psychological stress for women and men, and workplace and family stresses can spill over into each other. In two-job families, women often resent having a "double shift"—paid work plus housework—and men in turn feel that demands are made on them in the home that husbands in traditional marriages don't have (Glass and Fujimoto 1994). However, marriage extends men's and women's life spans, but through different means: "'His' marriage seems to consist of a settled life, improved perhaps by the household management skills and labors of his wife.... 'Her' marriage seems to offer primarily the benefits of improved financial well-being" (Lillard and Waite 1995: 1154).

The effects of workplace and family stress, role conflict, depression, and negative feelings on vulnerability to illness are hard to document. The connection between stress and heart attacks, for example, is not proven (Waldron 1995). Moreover, some "hardy personalities" thrive under stress (Ouellette 1993). A study of the effects of combined roles (work, marriage, and motherhood) in a sample of 1,473 Black and 1,301 White women found that work was significantly associated with lower blood pressure only for educated Black women (Orden et al. 1995). Being married was correlated with raised blood pressure for White women, but motherhood with lower blood pressure, even for single mothers.

Violence in Families

The home is not only a place of potential environmental hazards and stress, it can also be the site of physical violence, including murder. Although it is known to be seriously underreported, physical and sexual abuse by a family member affects millions of girls and women worldwide. According the World Health Organization, between 10 to 50 percent of women report being physically assaulted by an intimate partner in her lifetime.[17]

Men whose masculinity is tied to norms of dominance but who do not have the economic status to back up a dominant stance are likely to be abusive to the women they love, either psychologically or physically, and often both. James Ptacek's interviews with eighteen men in a counseling program for husbands who battered found that they felt they had a right to beat their wives: "There is a pattern of finding fault with the woman for not being good at cooking, for not being sexually responsive, for not being deferential enough ... for not knowing when she is 'supposed' to be silent, and for not being faithful. In short, for not being a 'good wife'" (1988, 147). Wife beating was once approved in most communities and is still condoned today where there is an ideology of men's authority over their wives. The response of the health professionals to emergency room visits by battered women indicates that many have ambivalent attitudes (Warshaw 1996).

Old Age: Women Live Longer but Not Better

Although the physiological aspects of old age seem to override social factors, in that women of every racial ethnic group in industrial societies outlive the men of their group, the quality of their lives in old age can suffer because of poverty and few social supports.

The later years of life present women and men with sex-specific health risks. The older men get, the more likely they are to develop prostate cancer, especially among Blacks (Weitz 1996, 53–55). It can be treated with surgery and chemotherapy, but both have side effects, such as impotence and urinary incontinence. After menopause, women are faced with increased risks of bone fragility and heart disease. In addition to these sex-specific physiological risks, social factors make getting older and dying different experiences for women and men. With longer life expectancy, many women in industrialized countries can expect to outlive their husbands or long-term male companions. As a result, an older woman will probably take care of the man she lives with during his last illness, but have no one to care for her when she is ill.[18] With the shift of convalescent care from hospitals to home, someone needs to give medications and injections and change wound dressings (Glazer 1990). Even if home health care givers are hired, someone needs to supervise and fill in; this "someone" is usually a wife or other woman relative. These caregivers frequently experience steady declines in their own physical and mental health throughout the duration of caregiving (Marks 1998).

For many elderly women, a daughter or daughter-in-law will help with shopping, housekeeping, and paying bills. But who takes care of elderly widows without children and those who have never married (Wu and Pollard 1998)? Women eighty-five years and older are more likely to be poor and living with relatives or in nursing homes than men of that age are (Longino 1988). Thus, for many women, the advantage of long life may not look like such a dividend after all.

Dying: Gendered Death Dips

One area in which social factors and physiological outcomes intertwine dramatically are "death dips." These are statistical drops in the expected rate of death in the weeks or days before a socially meaningful event, followed by a statistical rise a week or two later. Since the meanings of social events are gendered, we would expect that death dips would be, too. And so they are.

In the 1970s, David Phillips and his colleagues documented an intriguing epidemiological statistic—famous people were less likely to die in the month preceding their birthday than in the month after. He argued that they had postponed their deaths in order to participate in their public birthday celebrations. He also found, examining official tables of dates of death, that ordinary people also postponed dying until after important social occasions, such as presidential elections in the United States, and among Jews, the holiest day of the year, the Day of Atonement (Yom Kippur), and Passover, the popular celebration of liberation from Egyptian slavery (Phillips and Feldman 1973; Phillips and King 1988).

This and subsequent research has revealed that the death-dip phenomenon around major religious holidays is quite gendered, because of the different meanings of these events to women and men. Religious men tend to postpone death after major holidays that are centered on ritual observances; women tend to postpone death when the holidays are family-centered celebrations.

The Passover death-dip, for instance, occurs only among men. There was a 25.8-percent rise in deaths in the week after Passover among White men with unambiguously Jewish names who died in California between 1966 and 1984; for women, there was no such difference in deaths immediately before and after Passover (Phillips and King 1988). Although it is a family-centered holiday, the ritual seder is led by men; the cooking and serving is women's work. Statistical analysis of the death rates in a different population found the same gender pattern for all the major Jewish holidays (Idler and Kasl 1992). Jewish women's death patterns are similar to all nonobservant Jews—they are more likely to die in the month preceding a major holiday than in the month after, while Jewish men and all observant Jews are more likely to die in the month after (Idler and Kasl 1992, table 4).[19] These researchers' explanation is that Jewish men's involvement in religious observances is more central to their lives than to Jewish women, who are excluded from religious leadership in traditional Judaism.

The opposite pattern is true for Black and White Catholics and Protestants—women and men, observant and nonobservant, postpone death until after Christmas and Easter (Idler and Kasl 1992, table 3). In fact, women are more likely to postpone dying until after these events, which tend to be family-oriented rather than purely religious celebrations. A Finnish analysis of 60,000 deaths for the 1966–1986 period found that only women postponed dying until after Christmas, a family-centered holiday where the senior woman cooks the celebratory meal (Reunanen 1993).[20] A similar gendered phenomenon occurs around the Harvest Moon Festival among Chinese women aged seventy-five and older; their mortality rate is lower in the week before the holiday than in any other six-month period studied (Phillips and Smith 1990). Older women play the central part in the Harvest Moon Festival; the senior woman of the household supervises daughters and daughters-in-law in the preparation of an elaborate meal. The shift in dying does not occur among elderly Chinese men.

The dip in expected deaths the week before a major religious festival and the rise the week after has been documented for Chinese women with cerebrovascular and cardiac diseases and for Jewish men with these diseases and also with malignant tumors (Phillips and Smith 1990). Such psychosomatic and gendered effects of social beliefs are even starker among Chinese-Americans born in a year considered ill-fated in Chinese astrology who have a disease considered particularly detrimental for that birth year (Phillips et al. 1993). Their average age of death occurs almost two years earlier than among non-Chinese and those born in more advantageous years who have the same illnesses. Women with the ill-fated combination of birth year and disease lose more years of life than men. The gender pattern, the authors speculate, is due to greater traditionalism among Chinese-American women. However, the researchers argue that the crucial factors are behavior as well as beliefs. "Patients with ill-fated combinations of birth year and disease may refuse to change unhealthy habits because they believe their deaths are inevitable and thereby reduce their longevity. For example, earth patients with cancer may be less likely to quit smoking and fire patients with heart disease may be less likely to change their diets or exercise habits" (1993, 1144). How should a social epidemiologist classify these early deaths? Is the cause individual behavior, cultural beliefs, community practices, gender, ethnic identification, social class? Or all of the above?

Summary

Basic epidemiological statistics, such as life expectancy, cause of death, and illnesses throughout life, reflect the economic resources of a society, the levels of institutional racism, and the social status of women and men and girls and boys.

Women's longer life expectancy in modern industrialized societies depends in great part on access to medical care in pregnancy and childbirth. The effects of childbearing in adolescence, which often results in premature births and low birth-weight infants who may be physically underdeveloped, are associated with poverty, lack of prenatal care, and few social supports. When friends and family provide care and concern during pregnancies, the outcome is likely to be physically and psychologically favorable for both infants and mothers.

Hazardous work environments and delayed first pregnancies affect fetal development and sperm production and may result in infertility in men as well as women. In social stigma and extensiveness of treatment, however, the burden of infertility is much greater for women than for men. The constant innovation of assisted reproductive technologies as a means to achieve pregnancy is marketed to older, economically stable women.

From available data, we know that Black and Hispanic adolescents of both genders are more vulnerable to poor health and early death because they live in dangerous social environments, but girls and young women are less likely to engage in health-endangering behavior than boys and young men. Because of the combination of social factors in their disadvantaged neighborhoods and in their compensatory risk-defying actions, young Black and Hispanic men in United States inner cities have high rates of death from homicide, suicide, and accidents before they reach adulthood and from AIDS later on. Greater incarceration rates also expose disadvantaged young men to many health risks in prisons.

In adulthood, economic factors affect the health risks of women and men of various racial ethnic groups differently—poor men from disadvantaged groups are more vulnerable to occupational traumas and homicide; poor women from these groups to having and raising children in poverty. For all adults, smoking, drinking, taking drugs, lack of exercise, and poor diets are health-related behaviors somewhat under individual control, although having the time to exercise and the money to buy nutritional food may be significant situational obstacles to a healthy lifestyle. In addition, peer-group and family supports—social, psychological, and economic— influence individual health behaviors. These supports can be detrimental as well as protective, and their effects are gendered. Peer groups encourage alcohol consumption among college men and extreme forms of dieting among college women.

Juggling work and family responsibility may be more stressful for women than for men, but employment is beneficial to the physical and mental health of both women and men, providing not only income but a social circle. Having little control over one's work situation produces a high level of stress, so that people in low-level jobs and middle management may suffer more depression and psychosomatic illnesses than people in high positions. Men from disadvantaged racial ethnic groups and all women are most likely to have jobs with little mobility and autonomy. However, stress may not always be detrimental to health; some people have been found to thrive on it.

The home can also be the site of violence: Most women who are battered suffer at the hands of their husbands and lovers. A few fight back, and when they do, the violence escalates, often ending in homicide. The health care system does not often intervene in battering cycles, even when women show up in emergency rooms badly injured.

Old age and dying, like being born, are a gendered social phenomenon. Life expectancy and timing of death are influenced by social as much as physiological factors. Having someone to take responsibility for home care is as important as access to medical care in the longevity and quality of life of the elderly, and men are more likely to have a woman take care of them than vice versa.

The "death dip" phenomena, in which people with chronic or terminal illnesses postpone dying until after a meaningful event, such as a birthday, national election, or religious holiday, demonstrate the power of the social and psychological over physiology. The influence of gender is evident in the variable meaning of these events to different groups of women and men.

In sum, from the beginning to the end and throughout life, the human experiences of birth and death, disability and illness are embedded in social contexts. Because gender is such an important part of social life, women's and men's experiences, as we have seen, are different in sickness and in health, when rich and when poor, and in death, their lives are quite far apart.

Notes

1. "WHO Issues New Healthy Life Expectancy Rankings: Japan Number One in New 'Healthy Life' System." 2000. World Health Organization (WHO) Web site.

2. See note 1.

3. For the detrimental effects of extensive technology in childbirth, see Rothman 1986, 1989.

4. "UN Agencies Issue Joint Statement for Reducing Maternal Mortality." 1999. WHO Web site.

5. In India, the abuse of prenatal sex determination technologies for aborting female fetuses resulted in the 1996 law that criminalizes doctors, relatives, and the pregnant woman (Sudha and Rajan 1999). Despite the law, and condemnation by the Indian Medical Association and religious leaders of all faiths, the practices have continued in India and among émigrés in the United States (Sachs 2001).

6. See Abbey et al. 1991; Cooper and Glazer 1998; Sandelowski 1993; Spark 1988.

7. For discussions of the political and policy issues, see Merrick and Blank (1993).

8. Lesbian partners have used ART to ensure that both women have a biological relationship to the child. One partner's egg is inseminated with donor sperm, and the other partner gestates and gives birth (Sourbut 1997, 158).

9. National Vital Health Statistics Reports. 2000. CDC Web site.

10. Their lessened vulnerability to pregnancy and sexually transmitted diseases, however, is offset by their highly increased risk of traumatic injuries, such as torn knee ligaments, which girls seem to be particularly prone to (Longman 2001).

11. See note 9.

12. According to the DSM-IV, a diagnostic manual for mental health, more than 90 percent of anorexia cases are women.

13. "Anabolic Steroid Abuse." National Institute on Drug Abuse Research Report. 2000. NIDA Web site.

14. "Preliminary Results from the 1997 National Household Survey on Drug Abuse." 1998. Substance Abuse and Mental Health Services Administration (SAMHSA) Web site.

15. "Substance Abuse Treatment and Domestic Violence." 1997. SAMHSA Web site.

16. "Census of Fatal Occupational Injuries, 1998." U.S. Department of Labor Web site.

17. "Violence against Women." 2000. WHO Web site.

18. One study found that wives who become seriously ill and need care are vulnerable to divorce (James 2001).

19. Idler and Kasl did not break down their observant vs. nonobservant data by gender.

20. We are indebted to Elianne Riska for bringing this paper to our attention and for supplying us with an English summary and a description of Finnish Christmas customs.

CHAPTER 3

Hierarchies in Health Care:
Patients, Professionals, and Gender

I really don't know whether the influx of Blacks and women will change the medical profession in any fundamental way. The way medical education is, I think that sometimes there's a role that they want you to fill, and the pressures to conform to that role are so strong. There's a whole thing that if you're different, you're ostracized, you feel that you don't know as much. There have been some changes, but I don't know how widespread they're going to be. (Gamble 1982, 258)

Most people think of medicine as a man's profession, but the majority of the professional health care workers in Western medicine are women.[1] Women have been entering medical schools in the United States and Europe in greater numbers in the past thirty years. In the United States, women are 44 percent of medical students and 23 percent of all physicians.[2] In Finland, 49 percent of the professionally active doctors are women; in Sweden, 38 percent; in Denmark, 35 percent; and in Norway, 28 percent.[3] Despite their increasing numbers, the profession has not "feminized," but is still somewhat gender-segregated and gender-stratified. Men physicians tend to specialize in the more glamorous (and better-paying) areas, such as brain surgery, diseases of the heart, plastic surgery, and sports and space medicine; women physicians' specialties are primary care—family medicine, pediatrics, obstetrics and gynecology, dermatology, and ophthalmology—necessary but sometimes routinized work.

Since many women physicians work with other women health care professionals in clinics and primary care practices, patients more and more think of the health care provider as a woman (Coulter et al. 2000). In this chapter, we will look at the changing and continued hierarchies among health care professionals and the impact the growing number of women doctors has made on the delivery of health care.

Hierarchies of Health Care Providers

At the top levels of medical schools and research centers, women physicians are underrepresented compared to their numbers in the rest of the profession. More women than men have gone into academic medicine in the United States in recent years, but the "pipeline" leaks badly as they go up the professional ladder (Nonnemaker 2000). They are not promoted at the same rate as men doctors. Because women doctors still face sexism and lack effective mentors, they rarely become chiefs of departments or directors of major research centers, even if they are free of family obligations (Yedidia and Bickel 2001). In 1998, there were six women medical school deans out of 119 in the United States, with somewhat better representation as associate and assistant deans. However, three medical schools had no women deans at any level.[4]

The medical profession in the United States is imbalanced with regard to racial and ethnic groupings as well.[5] In 1999–2000, there were more African-American women medical students than men—3,188 to 2000, but more Asian/Pacific Islander men students than women—7,138 to 5,580. These were the two largest non-White groups in U.S. medical schools who were not foreign students. Compared to the 8 percent of medical students who were African American and the 19 percent who were Asian as of 1997, only 1 percent of the full professors were African American and 6 percent were Asian. There is only poor data on all physicians by racial and ethnic categorization.[6]

There are two main parallel health care professions—dentistry and pharmacy. The number of women dentists in the United States has doubled since 1987, from about 11,000 to more than 22,000 today, and they make up 28 percent of dentists under forty.[7] Currently, 19 percent of all dentists in the United States are women, but they are 31 percent of those who are professionally active. The majority, like men dentists, are in private practice. Only 4 percent specialize in pediatric dentistry. Despite their similarities, there are substantial gender differences in income and in teaching rank in dental schools. A comparison of women and men dentists in full-time general practice showed that men earn about $26,000 more per year than women dentists (Brown and Lazar 1998). The percentage of women dental school graduates has ranged between 35 and 38 percent since 1990; the percentage of women faculty in 1997 was 21.8 percent, of whom 6 percent were full professors, compared to 22 percent of the men faculty (AADS 1997). Thus, dentistry in the United States is still a man's profession, unlike many European countries, where it is considered women's work.

In the United States and Canada, more than half of pharmacists are women. In many European countries, it is a woman's profession. In North America, women pharmacists mainly work in hospitals or in chain stores, men as owners or managers of drugstores. The authors of a study of Canadian dentistry patterns feel that pharmacy is not feminizing; rather, it is quite gender-segregated by practice settings (Tanner and Cockerill 1996). However, in the United States, in nontraditional occupations for women, the workers with the highest median weekly earnings ($1,105) in 1999 were pharmacists; they earned more than women lawyers, electrical and electronic engineers, computer systems analysts and scientists, college and university teachers, and physical therapists.[8]

Nursing is the largest women's occupation in the United States, with two million registered nurses.[9] Most nurses work in hospitals, where they have increasing autonomy but ultimately take their orders from physicians. Their salaries range from $30,000 to $60,000, depending on region. Nurse practitioners work on their own or in clinics and do many of the examinations, vaccinations, and other primary care for minor illnesses, injuries, and checkups. They are licensed to prescribe medications. Other nurses with advanced degrees include certified nurse anesthetists and certified nurse-midwives. Among nurses in the United States, divisions are racial ethnic and class-based (Glazer 1991). Those in administration, teaching, and research are college-educated and predominantly White; licensed practical nurses and aids tend to be working-class women of color. Nursing aides, orderlies, and attendants number close to two million and 90 percent are women, many from disadvantaged groups and recent émigrées. In 2000, their median usual weekly earnings were $333; men in the same jobs earned 12 percent more.[10]

There has been a shortage of RNs in the United States for the past several years, with declining enrollments of students in entry-level bachelor's degree programs.[11] At the same time, enrollment for advanced nursing degrees and certificates has increased. These trends are not surprising, given the increased opportunities for women in medical and other professional schools, and the structural subordination of hospital nursing.

These gendered and racialized hierarchies of health care shape the encounters between patients and professionals.

Nurses: Doctor's Handmaidens or Partners?

Nursing has always been and still is a woman's profession. Women have always nursed the sick at home, and continue to do so, but since Florence Nightingale created nursing as part of medical care during the Crimean War at the end of the nineteenth century, women have supplied the hands-on care in hospitals and other medical settings.[12] There are men nurses and physicians' assistants (an occupation that grew out of military medics), but their numbers are small. Professional nursing's lack of attraction for men is in part the result of its history. Nightingale won doctors to the cause of professional nursing by making it clear that nurses would be "the physician's hand" and would only act under a doctor's orders. The schools she opened in Europe were for well-bred "gentlewomen"—middle-class women who wanted a genteel career. Almost like nuns, to this day in England nurses are called "sister," and the head nurse is called "matron."

In the United States, nursing schools were places where poor women could get room and board as well as training (Ashley 1976; Melosh 1982). Nursing schools were attached to hospitals—those for Black students to hospitals run by Black doctors to serve Black patients (Hine 1989). As students, nurses provided the hospitals to which their schools were attached with free labor; when they were sent out to do home nursing, their wages went to the school. As a result, when they graduated, they often could not find work, either in hospitals or as private nurses in homes. The road to unionization and good wages was long and hard (Sexton 1982). Today, nursing staffs are the first to be cut back when hospitals lose income because of lowered insurance payments. Many nurses have become an international mobile army of temporary and part-time workers, following personnel shortages.

Florence Nightingale succeeded in upgrading and professionalizing nursing through a curriculum that combined biomedical science with hygiene and hands-on bedside care. Everything the nurse did was to be medically therapeutic. When hospitalized patients' emotions and social situations were discovered in the mid-twentieth century to have an impact on their recovery rates, tender loving care (TLC) was added to nursing practice. In theory, the nurse was to be "mother" to the doctor "father," equally responsible for the patient "child." In practice, however, the nurses' job is to carry out the doctors' orders for medication, hooking up and watching machines, and monitoring vital signs (Strauss et al. 1985). If patients get any attention to their emotional needs, it is from women at the bottom of the hierarchy, such as nurses' aides and nursing home attendants, who are the lowest-paid paid health care workers (Diamond 1992).

Men nurses are encouraged by their mentors to move into positions of authority, as it is considered inappropriate for a man not to move up to supervisory and administrative positions. They are on a "glass escalator," upwardly mobile whether they are ambitious or not (Williams 1992). But they sometimes face a glass ceiling at higher levels. Women heads of nursing are too visible for them to be replaced by men.

Whether they are men or women, administrators or bedside caretakers, nurses' structural position in Western hospitals is subordinate to doctors, even when they work as a team. Nurses' training and practice is supposed to focus on care (contrasted with the physician's focus on cure), which "blurs the distinction between the medical and the social, the physiological and the psychological" (Fisher 1995, 10). Unfortunately, socioemotional care does not place very high in medical priorities. The doctor's perspective is the "voice of medicine"; the patient talks with the "voice of the lifeworld." These voices represent "the technical-scientific assumptions of medicine and the natural attitude of everyday life" (Mishler 1984, 14). Both voices need to be heard to understand an illness in its entirety, but, except for those doctors practicing medicine, the voice of medical authority usually prevails over the lifeworld voice of participating patients' experiences.

With the increase in women doctors, has this perspective changed?

Gender and Physicians' Practice Styles

The doctor-patient relationship is interactive, but the doctor usually sets the tone of the encounter. Today, men and women physicians both say they have to understand their patients' daily lives, work and family roles, and emotional needs to adequately treat them for physical illness, but patients claim that women physicians are more "humane"—more responsive to their social and emotional problems than men physicians (Fennema et al. 1990). These gender differences do not come from women doctors' motherliness or greater nurturance, but from the interactive and situational effects of the practice setting. As primary care physicians treating many aspects of the health problems of long-time patients, women physicians tend to encourage patients to participate by asking what they expect and think—and by listening to their answers. They talk more to their patients, but, more important, allow patients to talk more as well, especially about personal and family issues (Roter et al. 1991). In turn, patients feel that women doctors are less intimidating and so can be asked more questions and argued with (Roter and Hall 1998).

One study that found little difference in verbal communication between men and women physicians also found that women physicians' nonverbal communication styles were more supportive than those of men physicians (Hall et al. 1994). In comparing patients' behavior, they found that both men and women patients spoke more to women physicians and that women patients offered more medical information to women than to men physicians. The women physicians encouraged their women patients' narratives with supportive statements, "uh-huhs," and nodding. In contrast, the women physicians' interactions with men patients, who were usually older than they were, showed evidence of tension and role strain. In these encounters, older men patients' expectations that the doctor should be authoritative run counter to women doctors' egalitarian approach.

Participatory decision-making was the subject of a study of patients and physicians of different racial groups and genders (Cooper-Patrick et al. 1999). In telephone interviews, 1,816 patients of an urban managed care practice were asked to rate their primary care physicians on their participatory decision-making styles. The racial categories of the patients were 45 percent African American and 43 percent White; 66 percent were women. The 64 physicians who were evaluated were 25 percent African American, 56 percent White, and 37 percent were women. With all other variables held constant, patients whose racial category was the same as their physicians rated their visits as significantly more participatory than when they were of a different racial category. Women physicians were rated as more participatory in their decision-making than men physicians, but gender congruity was not a significant factor in patients' evaluations of the visit.

Gender congruity is a factor when lesbians who feel they will be stigmatized for their lifestyles seek out women physicians. Even if they are heterosexual, lesbian patients feel women doctors will be knowledgeable about their social situation because they have faced the same problems of sexual harassment and discrimination (Brogan et al. 1999). These concerns are recognized by health care professionals as well; for example, the U.S.

Institute of Medicine did a two-year study on the health care needs of lesbians (Solarz 1999).

In a study of health care encounters between lesbians and physicians, 45 lesbians, half of whom were women of color, evaluated 332 health care encounters with women and men doctors (Stevens 1996). In 92 percent of the accounts about men doctors, the women evaluated them negatively; the same was true for only 44 percent of the visits to women doctors. Negative aspects of care were "verbal intrusion on their dignity, denigration of their intellect, and dismissal of their concerns but also . . . loss of control over bodily appearance and reproductive functioning, violation of bodily safety, and sexualization" (p. 37). A positive encounter was characterized by what was described as "solidarity: compassionate competence, empowering information exchange, and negotiated action" (p. 29). Particularly valued was "pragmatic clinical competence [combined with] sympathetic consciousness of clients' needs" (p. 29), so that medical advice was offered in a way appropriate to the client's situation. The lesbian clients wanted knowledge that would enable them to promote and maintain their own health and well-being, and they also appreciated being involved in the diagnosis and decisions about treatment.

Because so many women doctors are in primary care, patients come to them with all their problems—major and minor illnesses, physical and emotional symptoms. There is a danger, then, that they will become "the defacto psychosocial experts in the care of patients and increasingly assume responsibility for the management of emotionally distressed patients" (Roter and Hall 1998, 1096). This expertise can have a backlash. Doctors of either gender in office practice generally prefer similar types of patients—those who allow them to carry out their work with a minimum of fuss, who are cooperative, trusting, appreciative, and responsive to treatment (Lorber 1984, 56–57). In one study, however, more women doctors said they liked their patients than men doctors did (Hall et al. 1993). The differences patients perceive between men and women doctors may be a self-fulfilling prophecy. If patients think women doctors are more empathic, the women may in turn cultivate an expressive style to meet patients' expectations. Thus, women doctors may or may not be more attuned to the "whole patient" because they are women, but if patients think they are, they may prefer a woman doctor, especially for primary care. However, they may also be more dissatisfied with their care if a woman doctor does not live up to their gendered expectations. Patient-centered skills can be taught in medical schools, and it would be better for patients if men as well as women doctors learned to use them and to make them part of their general routine (Roter and Hall 1998).

Are Women Doctors Better for Women Patients?

When we look at medical practice, we find that not only do women and men doctors have different practice styles, but that women doctors order more tests for women patients.[13]

In an area of medical practice where the risks for women are well known—breast and cervical cancer—as are the guidelines for regular Pap smears and mammograms, whether they are recommended seems to depend on the gender of the doctor. Studies covering thousands of patients in the United States have found large, statistically significant differences between the recommendations for these tests by women and men doctors. In one study using a national sample of 5,536 women patients, the more than 90 percent with men health care providers were less likely than those with women doctors to have had a Pap test in the previous three years, and for those over age forty-five, to ever have had a mammogram (Franks and Clancy 1993).

Another study, which used the records of a large midwestern medical health plan, found that women who were patients of women doctors were nearly twice as likely to have received a Pap test and 40-percent more likely to have had a mammogram the previous year than women who had seen a doctor who was a man (Lurie et al. 1993). The researchers analyzed the claims for Pap smears and mammograms of 27,713 women patients who had seen only one doctor the previous year for the gender, age, and specialty of that doctor. The doctors were in internal medicine and family practice (550) and obstetrics-gynecology (130). Twenty percent of all of these doctors were women, and they were on average about ten years younger than the men doctors. Among the gynecologists, the younger men doctors (38 to 42 years old) were less likely than all the women and the older men to order cancer-screening tests. Among the internists and family practitioners, the men doctors ordered significantly fewer of these tests than the women doctors, with those under 38 years old having the lowest rates of all. The authors of this study questioned why, among younger doctors, whose medical education has stressed the need for preventive screening, men are so reluctant to recommend Pap smears and mammograms to their women patients. They argued that perhaps these tests were easier to discuss when the doctor and patient were of the same gender. However, such reluctance in men who are gynecologists is disturbing.

A study that focused on family practitioners added cholesterol testing—a gender-neutral area (Kreuter et al. 1995). The researchers interviewed women patients in twelve family practices in North Carolina, 1,630 whose regular provider was one of thirty-three men doctors, and 220 who usually saw one of five women doctors. They found that among the patients older than twenty years who had not had a cholesterol test in five years, those seeing a woman doctor were 56 percent more likely to get the test than those seeing a man.

In short, women patients are more likely to get good preventive care if they have a woman doctor than if they have a doctor who is a man. The increasing focus on women's health as a specialized body of knowledge is likely to increase this gap, if it is not integrated into the medical school curriculum (Nicolette and Jacobs 2000). At present, the "women's health physician" seems to be emerging as a new specialist without much altering the overall outlook or structure of Western health care. As Elianne Riska says in her assessment of women's health advocacy, "The women's health physician serves as an advocate for women's health needs as well as an expert and feminist promoter of medical knowledge on women's health" (2001, 143). Unlike the feminist criticism of male biases in Western biomedicine that burgeoned in the 1980s, the current perspective of women's health physicians and researchers is integrative (Pinn 2001).

There is certainly a recognition of women patients' health needs in the major medical journals, but the continued viability of the Women's Health Initiative in the U.S. National Institutes of Health and professional journals dedicated to the topic indicate that women are still considered separate and different—and not the norm (Harrison 1990).

Can Women Doctors Change Health Care?

How much of an impact has the recent influx of women doctors had on medicine as a whole? Has their presence made a difference, or have they assimilated the standard biomedical biases and perspectives? These questions have been raised as Western medicine seems to be "going female" in the United States as well as in other countries.[14] Not only will women physicians have a quantitative majority, but the new generation is coming into a changed profession, one where the power and prestige of the physician depends less on charismatic authority than on the ability to command organizational resources for research and practice.

The status and influence of women doctors is dependent on the organization and financing of health care, which underpin the authority and autonomy of physicians in the medical division of labor (Riska 2001). In capitalist countries before World War II, doctors were usually solo, fee-for-service practitioners, with sole authority over their patients. In Europe first, and then in the United States, medicine has become more regulated and paid for by governments or an expanding insurance industry. As it became a profession where the doctor's authority was diluted and income has decreased, medicine has lost its attractiveness for men, leaving an occupational niche for women. Until now, despite their increasing numbers, women doctors have not become a substantial proportion of the medical leadership. A combination of institutionalized and informal practices have steered them into primary care and family practice. When they did go into academic medicine and research, they were not usually mentored by senior men doctors for positions of authority. As a result, even in countries where women have been the majority of doctors, the top positions in large medical centers, medical schools, and research centers have been held predominantly by men. These institutions develop medical knowledge, decide what medical students are taught, and determine standard practices for diagnosis and treatment. If women physicians are to make a significant impact on the delivery of services or the production and dissemination of medical knowledge, they will have to be sponsored by senior men for high-level administrative positions as chiefs of service in hospitals, deans of medical schools, and directors of large research centers (Freidson 1986). That is, senior men have to be willing to encourage women to be their replacements when they retire.

What do women physicians bring to health care that is different? They have a history of attention to the psychosocial needs of patients. In the United States in the nineteenth century, women doctors specialized in the health care of women and children, set up their own clinics and hospitals, and incorporated social needs into their services (Drachman 1984; Morantz-Sanchez 1985). The maternity clinics, for example, attended to the social difficulties of unmarried mothers. Gloria Moldow's (1987) history of Black and White women doctors in Washington, D.C., at the end of the nineteenth century describes medical communities segregated by race and gender. White women doctors set up their own infirmaries when they were denied access to the dispensaries and clinics that gave novice White men doctors clinical experience and contacts. The women doctor's infirmaries were run for mostly women and children patients, and offered free and low-cost care. Only the Woman's Clinic, which was completely staffed by women, including a Black woman doctor, survived the rise of the scientifically oriented, better-equipped university hospitals, which became, in Moldow's words, "no-woman's land." Through federal funding, Black men had Howard Medical School and tax-supported hospitals to work in, but few of the Black women doctors were able to attract enough patients to practice medicine full-time; many taught science in segregated high schools (Moldow 1987, 129–33).

Darlene Clark Hine's description of the lives and work of the 115 Black women who became doctors in late-nineteenth-century America after slavery was abolished shows that many founded hospitals, nursing schools, and social service agencies as adjuncts to their private practices because none were available for the Black patients in their communities, especially in the South (1985). They were important members of their communities—as professionals, as daughters of prominent families, and as wives of ministers, educators, and fellow doctors.

After World War I, when women got the vote in the United States, they helped to pass the Sheppard-Towner Act, which, in 1921, set up state and federally funded maternal and child health centers throughout the country (Muncy 1991). These centers were staffed by women doctors and social workers, and they offered free medical services and preventive care. They also propagandized for the medicalization of childbirth and delivery by obstetricians, not midwives. By 1929, in the face of the desperate need of its members for paying patients during the Depression, the American Medical Association, dominated by men in solo, fee-for-service practice, led the fight to deny further funding to the Sheppard-Towner clinics.

In the 1960s, when Medicare and Medicaid increased the numbers of patients, the doors of U.S. medical schools and hospitals opened to women. Few women doctors determined curriculum; physician professors and senior residents were mostly men, and training paid little attention to the social situations of men or women patients (Harrison 1983; Scully 1994). Many of the women students followed the recommendations of their men advisors and went into obstetrics and gynecology and family practice, and in time became advocates for women's health care.

In the 1970s in the United States, the feminist health movement established client-run clinics for women patients that stressed education in health matters, gynecological self-examination, and alternative medicines. Their goal was to take the control of women's bodies out of the hands of the medical system, because they felt it was male-dominated and oppressive (Ruzek 1978). The problem women patients faced, according to the feminist health movement, was two-fold: a system that allowed patients very little control over their own health care, and biomedical knowledge and practices that ignored many of women's life circumstances. The cause, they argued, was a body of knowledge and clinical practices dominated by White middle-class men and their values. In medical textbooks, men's bodies were the norm; women's bodies deviations from the norm (Scully and Bart 1973). Menstruation, childbirth, and menopause were considered illnesses instead of part of women's normal life cycle (Martin 1992). Gynecological and obstetric practices could be brutal (Rothman 1982; Scully 1994). Doctors gave women patients too little information and rarely consulted them about their wishes before ordering hysterectomies and other drastic treatment (Fisher 1986; Todd 1989).

Although the feminist clinics preferred women to men doctors for their legally required medical backup, they were not trusted any more than men doctors, because both had been trained in the same masculinist biomedical curriculum. The activists in the feminist health movement thought that by educating women patients to be more assertive and knowledgeable health consumers, they would put pressure on medical schools to modify the way doctors were taught to practice.

The feminist health movement, the influx of women doctors into obstetrics and gynecology, and the resurgence of midwives did change how pelvic examinations were done and made childbirthing more participatory and family-oriented. However, there are still significant differences between midwives, who have a more holistic approach to pregnancy and childbirth, and obstetricians, whose focus is on pathology (Rothman 1982).

By the 1990s, most of the feminist health movement's general clinics had been abandoned (Ruzek and Becker 1999). The consumer movement in health care had enormously strengthened all patients' rights to question their care, but they still had to get that care through a doctor-dominated system (Haug and Lavin 1983). Family practice and other primary care specialties (obstetrics and gynecology, pediatrics, gerontology) have had an influx of resources in the United States. These general practitioners are the main workers in hospital outpatient clinics, health maintenance organizations, managed care, and other settings where services are paid for by insurance plans or the government. As the numbers of women in medical school have increased, they have been encouraged to go into these burgeoning specialties and into primary care settings. Whether that makes for care more oriented to patients' needs depends on whether doctors whose approach is the whole patient are able to structure their time to deliver holistic health care. As primary care providers in group practice or clinic settings, women physicians have a fixed amount of time to spend with patients (Riska 1993). They may not be in a position to structure their delivery of health care to be sensitive to patients unless they are in their own solo or small group practices (Candib 1995).

Women physicians' efforts have made women's health care needs more visible in the profession as a whole. In the last few years, women doctors in the United States have promoted research and held conferences on women's diverse health needs. A workshop held in 1997 called for participatory research based on "women's experience, both of their physiology and of their psychosocial, home, and work environments" (Harlow et al. 1999). Another recommendation was to look beyond the Western world for data on women's health. Medical journals for women doctors have published articles on health care for women with disabilities and lesbians, and discussed human rights issues, such as female genital surgery and politically motivated rape.

When she was director of the National Institutes of Health, Dr. Bernadine Healy set up an Office of Women's Health Research and began a Women's Health Initiative. She said that the reason she did so was not only to study the illnesses that affect women alone, but to look at gender differences in illnesses that affected women as well as men, such as heart disease. These have been researched with men subjects, and only when the woman patient's symptoms emulated those of a man was she treated adequately. Healy called this problem "the Yentl syndrome" after the fictional nineteenth-century Jewish girl who disguised herself as a man in order to attend school and study the Talmud (Healy 1991).

Even if women doctors did run medicine as they do nursing, there is little indication that they would make care less biomedical and technological (Todd 1989, 101–29). Biochemistry and pathology of the body are the current bases of Western medical knowledge. Women and men doctors who believe that social, environmental, family, and psychological concerns should be an integral part of medical knowledge are not likely to restructure Western biomedicine unless medical school curricula and training include this information (Dan 1994). Until the model of care is socio-biomedical, "medicine remains the real stuff of clinical practice unsullied by social concerns" (Fisher 1995, 202).

Summary

Women are most of the health care workers in Western medicine, and they are approaching the majority of doctors as well. Their numbers and their organized efforts have begun to make medical practice and medical research more responsive to the health care needs of women. Two parallel professions, dentistry and pharmacy, vary in the number of women and men. In the United States, these professions are men's work; in other countries, they are women's work.

In the organization of Western health care, most of the doctors who are in positions of power—heads of medical schools, hospitals, and large research centers—have been men, with women doctors mostly in primary care. Women physicians' first-hand medical practices and more egalitarian practice styles are attuned to patients' psychosocial needs. They have developed patient-oriented communication styles that can be taught to other doctors. Women physicians who have been in a position to change training programs and develop doctor-patient protocols on women's health for widespread use have substantially altered medical school curricula.

Nurses are mostly women, and their training and practice emphasizes care—attention to the patient's psychosocial as well as biomedical needs. In hospitals, however, nurses take orders from doctors. A coalition of women physicians and women nurses has the potential to make the delivery of health care more patient-oriented.

Women doctors, like nurse practitioners, talk more to their patients about psychosocial issues and their concerns about their illness, and also offer patients more opportunities to question and argue. These differences in communication styles make women doctors seem more humane than men doctors, and preferred for primary care, since "patients clearly favor doctors who engage them personally through social conversation, who use positive language, who use partnership language, who acknowledge the patient's emotions, who discuss psychological problems, and who behave in an interested, friendly, and responsive overall manner" (Hall and Roter 1995, 91). The latent effect, however, is to reinforce the gendered stratification of health practitioners, with women in direct, hands-on, first-line care, and men in prestigious and powerful administrative and policy-making positions.

A transformed Western health care system would put more emphasis on patients' emotional and social needs and also give patients more autonomy in making decisions about their treatment. Whether women doctors in positions of power make these changes depends on whether they adopt the standard biomedical outlook of the profession or critique it, as feminists have done. The basis of Western medicine is physiology and biology; social and environmental aspects of illness are secondary concerns. In addition, health professionals are the experts and so their determination of the cause and treatment of the patient's ailments is likely to prevail over the patient's view of what she or he needs. A gender-integrated health care system is not likely to be much different from what we have today unless women physicians use their prestige to challenge and modify it.

NOTES

1. Women comprise almost 80 percent of the U.S. health care work force, according to the U.S. Department of Labor Bureau of Labor Statistics, January 1999.

2. Data on U.S. women physicians are from the Women in Medicine Data Source on the American Medical Association's Web site.

3. Nordic Medical Associations Web site, 1999 data.

4. See note 2.

5. Data are from the Minority Physicians' Data Source on the American Medical Association's Web site.

6. As of the end of 1998, the AMA had race/ethnicity data on about 60 percent of all physicians and 51 percent for all women physicians in the United States.

7. Data on women dentists are from the Web sites of the American Women's Dental Association, the American Dental Association, the Chicago Dental Society, and the Women's Bureau of the Department of Labor.

8. Women's Bureau, U.S. Department of Labor Web site: "20 Leading Occupations of Employed Women, 2000 Annual Averages."

9. Data on nurses in the United States are from the American Nursing Association Web site. Statistics are based on 1992 and 1996 surveys.

10. See note 6.

11. Data are from the Association of American Nursing College's annual survey of 2000 summary on the AANC Web site.

12. For histories of nursing after Florence Nightingale, see Ashley 1976, Hine 1989, Melosh 1982, Reverby 1987.

13. None of the studies discussed in this section report on racial ethnic breakdowns of physicians or patients.

14. See Lorber 1984, Notzer and Brown 1995, Pringle 1998, Riska 2001, Riska and Wegar 1993a.

CHAPTER 4

Gender and Disability:
Contradictions and Status Dilemmas

Whoever I was, whatever I had, there was always a sense that I should be grateful to someone for allowing it to happen, for like women, I, a handicapped person, was perceived as dependent on someone else's largesse for my happiness, or on someone else to *let* me achieve it for myself. (Zola 1982a, 213)

Because disability involves physical and sensory functioning, it may be difficult to think of the status of "disabled" as socially constructed, but as with illness, it is deeply shaped by social contexts.[1] Whether physically or sensorally challenged people can work at paid jobs and care for themselves and others depends to a great extent on the availability of technological devices, transportation, and the physical environment, but perhaps more on the active participation of employers, families, and friends.

The U.S. Census Bureau's definition of *disability* is "difficulty . . . seeing, hearing, talking, walking, climbing stairs and lifting and carrying" or "doing school work for children, working at a job or around the house for adults."[2] A person who cannot perform one or more activities, uses an "assistive device to get around, or who needs assistance from another person to perform basic activities is considered to have a severe disability." Based on this definition, one in five Americans has a disability and one in ten a severe disability. About 9 million people need personal assistance to carry out everyday activities; 80 percent of these helpers are relatives, nearly half of whom live with the person with a disability. As people get older, they are more likely to have a disability, but racial ethnic status is also a factor. For those aged 55 to 64, 20 percent of Whites, 29 percent of those of Hispanic origin, and 35 percent of Blacks had a severe disability in the late 1990s.

Despite this broad definition of disability, legal benefits are tied to employability. In the United States, what qualifies a worker for disability compensation depends on "what is expected of the nondisabled—what injuries, diseases, incapacities, and problems they will be expected to tolerate in their normal working lives" (Stone 1984, 4). Only if the inability to work goes beyond these "normal" incapacities is the person considered disabled. Qualifying for Social Security Disability Income in the United States involves having been gainfully employed for at least five of the ten years preceding the disability and to be unable any longer to work at a paid job (Reisine and Fifield 1988). Other retirement systems for the permanently disabled are similarly tied to previous waged occupations (Stone 1984). Homemakers who can no longer do housework or childcare have no way of providing money to hire someone who can replace their essential work for their families.

Within the last decade, the social status of people with disabilities has changed in ways reflected in that very designation—they are people first, not "the handicapped" or "the disabled," which erases their personhood. Yet the designation of "people with disabilities" constitutes a *status dilemma*—in the eyes of able-bodied people, physical incapacities devalorize whatever else they accomplish.[3] People with disabilities have been able to assert their competence and capabilities in their work and family lives, but their status gets undercut by the negative attributes still attached to their physical disabilities. This status dilemma has often been handled by keeping coping strategies and physical helps under cover—what sociologists call "deviance disavowal" (Davis 1972). For example, Bob Dole, who has little control over his right arm, always clutches a pen in his right hand to keep the fingers from splaying. When he campaigned for the presidency of the United States in 1996, his right side was protected from crowds by his aids, and they unobtrusively gave him a pad to lean on when he signed autographs (Kelly 1996). In such encounters among people of different physical capabilities, interaction proceeds as if everyone were on the same footing. But the person who does not have the full use of limbs, eyes, ears, voice, or other bodily functions knows how much effort goes into making it possible to participate socially as an equal.

When we introduce the factor of gender, the social situation of the person with disabilities becomes an even more complex status dilemma. A man who wants to present himself as masculine needs to have an aura of independence, even when he relies on the help of others. A woman who wants to present herself as feminine may end up seeming helpless and fragile, undercutting her presentation of herself as an independent adult.

For men, in order to maintain a high status, disabilities have had to be rendered invisible or transformed into heroism. Franklin Delano Roosevelt, a polio victim who served as president of the United States from 1932 to 1944, masked his inability to walk or to stand without supports (Gallagher 1985). John Hockenberry, a paraplegic due to an automobile accident, has gone around the world as a reporter in his wheelchair, admittedly flaunting his physical state (Hockenberry 1995). Although disabilities are now more visible, they are still not completely accepted. Perhaps the unremarked presence in a wheelchair of President Bill Clinton's impressive counsel, Charles Ruff, at the drawn-out impeachment trials of 1998–1999, will go far toward normalizing disabilities in the public eye.

While men with disabilities try to project masculine strength, women with disabilities have also used overcoming adversity to enhance their self-image. Some women have reported feeling more capable and attractive in a wheelchair than on crutches (Lonsdale 1990, 69–70). Nancy Mairs says she prefers to consider herself a cripple, rather than disabled or handicapped: "People—crippled or not—wince at the word 'cripple,' as they do not at 'handicapped' or 'disabled.' Perhaps I want them to wince. I want them to see me as a tough customer, one to whom the fates/gods/viruses have not been kind, but who can face the brutal truth of her existence squarely. As a cripple, I swagger" (1986, 9). Mairs' presentation of self is "tough," a stance for women or men who want to confront the world on their own terms, like Diana Golden Brosnihan.

Many people with disabilities are heroes in their everyday lives, but for the more able-bodied public, physically disabled athletes are the stars—at least while they are newsworthy. The death from cancer on August 25, 2001, of Diana Golden Brosnihan at age thirty-eight brought renewed attention to "a remarkable life" (Araton 2000, D1). Diana Golden was a skier when she was five years old. She developed bone cancer when she was twelve, and she resumed skiing six months after her right leg was amputated above the knee. Skiing on one leg with regular ski poles, she competed against two-legged skiers and won a gold medal in the giant slalom in the 1988 Winter Olympics, as well as ten world and nineteen U.S.

championships from 1986 to 1990, skiing against others with disabilities (Litsky 2001). She married Steve Brosnihan, a cartoonist, in 1997, while she was undergoing chemotherapy for a recurrence of cancer.

Golden Brosnihan was always unhappy with her status dilemma as "disabled athlete." She didn't want to be admired because she had overcome a disability. "She wanted admiration for her technique, her skill, for how she had discarded disabled ski equipment for regular ski poles to produce faster times and fought successfully to compete in the same races with the nonhandicapped" (Araton 2001, D1). In recognition of her fight for equal status, her citation when she was inducted into the Women's Sports Foundation International Hall of Fame in 1997 read, "She persuaded the ski world to treat all athletes the same, regardless of ability or, in her case, disability" (Litsky 2001).

Gender Contradictions in Disability

In a widely cited paper, Michelle Fine and Adrienne Asch (1985) argued that women with disabilities face "sexism without the pedestal." Compared to men of a similar level of physical functioning, they are less likely to find jobs that allow them to be economically independent. They are also less likely to have a lifetime partner, because they need the care and attention that women are expected to give to others, although they may be better able to find a life partner or a circle of women caregivers if they are lesbian.[4] Heterosexual women with disabilities, however, may find the fulfillment of traditional wife-mother gender roles beyond reach.

The opposite situation occurs for men with disabilities, who are more likely to find a life partner. In the traditional husband role, care received is recompensed with economic support, so as long as a man with disabilities can earn an income, he can fulfill his family role obligations. Sexuality and its machismo qualities are particularly devastating minefields for men with disabilities, but it is also a problem for men who have had prostate surgery and older men. Indeed, the immense popularity of Viagra seems to indicate that actual or imagined sexual dysfunction is practically pandemic among men. In short, despite the conventional wisdom that "'disabled man' is a self-contradiction, because men are stereotypically supposed to be 'able,' strong, and powerful" (Lakoff 1989, 368), a man with disabilities may be quite able to function well as a husband, father, and lover.

There is a loop-back effect between gender and disability. Family and work roles are gendered, and these affect the expectations for a person with disabilities. In turn, being a woman or a man with permanent disabilities modifies work opportunities, living arrangements, family life, friendships, intimate relationships, and a person's sense of self (Charmaz 1995). The actual lived experience of women and men with disabilities often contradicts the stereotypes of both gender and disability. However, the behavior of families, professional caretakers, and physicians toward people with disabilities is more likely to reflect conventional ideas of what women and men should be. What the person with disabilities wants and can accomplish is encouraged or discouraged according to beliefs about "normal" gendered behavior.

The influence of gender expectations on caregiving and the socialization of children with a disability is clearly illustrated by a study of 32 low-income African-American mothers of sons and daughters with sickle cell anemia (Hill and Zimmerman 1995). The children ranged in age from 2 months to 22 years, with an average age of 10.4 years. Through in-depth interviews, the researchers found that the mothers of daughters encouraged normal activities, including physical exertion, a stoical attitude toward minor symptoms, and self-care. In contrast, the mothers of sons described them as "fragile, certainly too fragile to conform to the traditional male gender role. The mothers tried to protect their sons from excessive physical activity, especially participation in sports" (p. 47). The mothers of sons with symptomatic sickle cell anemia were less likely to work outside the home than the mothers of daughters with the same level of functioning. They were more likely to do all they could to prevent their sons from suffering crises of pain and inability to breathe. In short, sickle cell anemia was not seen by these African-American mothers as preventing their daughters' growing up to be competent women, but was seen for their sons as "requiring behavior at odds with the aggressiveness, risk taking, and physical activity of the male gender role" (p. 48). As a result, the mothers of daughters treated them the way they would any girl child, but the mothers of sons treated them as especially "vulnerable and in constant danger" (p. 48).

This study shows that caregivers start with an ideal of how women and men should behave and then do an assessment of whether the person with disabilities can live up to that ideal. If the assessment is that the person cannot, then the means of living normally are denied. The outcome reinforces the gendered expectations rather than providing alternative ways of being a woman or a man. The content of the gender expectations is not the issue—beliefs that women can take care of themselves or need protection, that men have to be physically assertive or are characterized by their earning ability vary by culture and social group. It is the power of the assumptions and their translation into behavioral expectations for people with disabilities that create dual constraints for women and men who are especially dependent on others for personal care and emotional support.

Gendered Caregiving

The mainstreaming of people with disabilities depends on access to technological devices and on personal caregivers, who are often women family members. Women have nursed sick family members as a longstanding part of their work as mothers, daughters, and grandmothers. As professional and informal caregivers, women are the majority of the nurses and health care workers in hospitals and nursing homes, and in the home. Because it so closely resembles socially appropriate work for women, care is usually done by women for women and men. Men with disabilities are more likely to be economically self-supporting and therefore more likely to have a wife to take care of their physical and emotional needs than women with disabilities, who are less likely to have a lifetime partner to look after them. They have to support themselves economically, and also fend for themselves physically and emotionally. They may even end up taking care of others.

A study of twenty-five middle-aged women with a variety of disabilities (blindness, hearing loss, polio, spinal cord injuries, cerebral palsy, rheumatoid arthritis, and multiple sclerosis), who needed help with daily activities, nevertheless "nurtured children, spouses, other family members, co-workers, and pets" (Quinn and Walsh 1995, 243). In a review of the autobiographies of twenty-five blind and visually impaired women and men, Adrienne Asch and Lawrence Sacks found that a common theme was that of the "self-sacrificing, supportive, nurturing mother" (1983, 244). The men had one; the women became one. In adulthood, few of the women with visual impairments married, and most chose careers in teaching, social work, and rehabilitation; the men attained high status in business or professions and married sighted women. Asch and Lawrence conclude that "the women provided support, warmth, and love for blind people just as their mothers did for them as blind children. The men . . . tended to marry replicas of their mothers, whereas the women [symbolically] became their mothers" (1983, 244).

When women care for husbands with disabilities, they are doing what wives ordinarily do, only more extensively. A wife's attentiveness to a husband's needs, Kathy Charmaz points out, validates the centrality of his position in the household (1995). For men, caregiving is not the usual part of the husband or father role. As Robert Murphy, physically dependent on his wife because of a progressive spinal tumor, says: "Husbands become part-time nurses, which goes against social conventions, and wives find themselves with an additional child, which doesn't" (1990, 206).

Yet the demands of caregiving are not gender-specific. Caregiving is a difficult combination of physical and emotional work—lifting, turning, toileting, feeding, bathing, clothing, encouraging, calming, hugging, kissing, talking (Corbin and Strauss 1988). Barbara Hillyer, reflecting on her care for her daughter, notes that "caring requires that exceptional physical and emotional strength be exercised. . . . The . . . caregiver is expected to be available, dependable, and constant," well-organized, empathic, but not expectant of emotional responsiveness from the recipient of care (1993, 11). It is the compatibility of caregiving duties with gendered family roles that makes it seem as if women are "natural" home nurses.

Women may be the designated caregivers, but they often find the burdens as difficult as men do. One study of spousal care gave quotes from eight wives and two husbands—the wives described excessive physical work, guilt feelings, hiding their worries, drinking too much, being constantly nervous, depressed, or devastated; one husband talked of his resentment when he came home from work to a sick wife, the other of his sexual deprivation (Corbin and Strauss 1988, 289–317). In one dramatic case, a caregiving husband, George Delury, age sixty-two, helped his fifty-two-year-old wife, Myrna Lebove, commit suicide with a drink of antidepressants, water, and honey that he had mixed for her. They had been married after she developed her first symptoms of multiple sclerosis and had been together for twenty-two years. When her physical and mental condition deteriorated badly, Mr. Delury started a diary entitled "Countdown: a Daily Log of Myrna's Mental State and View toward Death." In it, he said that he had four options—abandon his wife, keep taking care of her and go mad, kill himself, or kill her. On the evidence of the diary, he was indicted for manslaughter, pleaded guilty, and was sentenced to six months in prison (Goldberg 1995; Pierre-Pierre 1996).

Although women are more likely to be family caregivers than men are, there is ample evidence of men competently and willingly taking care of physically and mentally impaired relatives—women as well as men.

A survey of a national sample of 233 mostly Caucasian men caregivers age thirty-six to eighty-four showed that, although they had not been socialized for the work, they were able to learn "on the job." The majority were caring for women with Alzheimer's disease. Like fathers who share parenting duties and single fathers of young children, men caregivers develop skills and empathy (Applegate and Kaye 1993). They are, however, less likely to be competent in the routinized supervisory and concrete tasks that are so typical of "women's work":

> In contrast to the stereotype that male caregiving is primarily instrumental in nature, these men's responses suggested that, overall, the tasks associated with social support were those they performed most frequently, most competently, and with the greatest degree of satisfaction. Ranked second in degree of frequency, competence, and level of satisfaction were instrumental daily living tasks, followed by case management tasks and, in last place, the "hands-on" functional aspects of personal care. (Kaye and Applegate 1990, 84)

The reluctance of the men in this study to handle a woman's body may be because many were caring for mothers. We would need more detailed accounts by men of their care of fathers, mothers, wives, and children of different ages and genders to have the full range of their caregiving activities among family members.[5] Outside of families, there is a great deal of evidence of the caregiving and emotional and social support of men to men ill with AIDS (Turner et al. 1993).

Gender and Altruism

When wives and mothers care for family members with disabilities, they are expanding already existing roles. But altruism seems to imbue women's overall behavior more than it does men's responses to calls to give. The gender effects evident in caregiving are highlighted in an extreme form of altruistic behavior—donation of a kidney to a relative with chronic renal disease. For the person who needs a kidney transplant, a successful donation means freedom from dialysis and, in many cases, survival. About 70 percent retain the kidney, and their subsequent physical and psychological quality of life is good (Simmons et al. 1987, xxii–xxiii). The cost to the donor is loss of a healthy kidney with risk of subsequent failure of the remaining kidney, surgery with general anesthesia, at least a week's hospitalization with consequent loss of stamina, and an extensive abdominal scar. The risk of the operation to a donor's life is calculated at 0.05 percent and the long-term risk at 0.07 percent (Simmons et al. 1987, 39, 165–75).

Studies of gender differences in live kidney donors found that wives are much more likely to donate a kidney to a husband than vice versa (Zimmerman et al. 2000). Among spouses, 36 percent of wives who were acceptable donors went on to donate, compared with only 6.5 percent of acceptable husbands. Women in general are less likely to be ambivalent about donating a kidney to a relative with end-stage renal disease than men are (Simmons et al. 1987, 188–89). Mothers asked to donate a kidney to a child are more likely to be free of doubt than fathers (58 percent to 29 percent), and sisters are more likely than brothers to be sure about their decision to donate (56 percent to 28 percent). Daughters agreeing to donate to a parent are surer that they are doing the right thing than are sons (27 percent to 11 percent).

After the kidney has been donated, men have more negative feelings than women do about what they have undergone, and these feelings persist a year later. However, men are more likely to feel better about themselves immediately post-transplant (23 percent to 8 percent of women donors) and one year later (40 percent to 26 percent), indicating that the women's donation may have been taken more for granted as part of their duty *as women*. The authors surmise that these gender differences are due to women's and men's experiences as actual or potential parents:

> Perhaps donation seems to the female to be a simple extension of her usual family obligations, while for the male it is an unusual type of gift. . . . Giving birth to an infant is congruent psychologically with the act of giving a body-part so a loved one can be reborn. . . . From a male's point of view, there is no life experience or expectation like childbirth that prepares him for this act of donation. Thus he may have stronger ambivalences and doubts even after the transplant. In any case, whether his feelings are positive or negative, he is more likely to feel he has performed an exceptional act. If his feelings are positive, as the majority of men's are, he is more likely to reap self-image benefits from this extraordinary gift. (pp. 188–89)

In this sense, women's bodily sacrifice is that of a "normal, natural" mother; men's image is similar to what is fostered when they are wounded in battle. They are heroes.[6]

A Man but Not a Man, a Woman but Not a Woman

Gendering of people with disabilities is especially evident in sexuality and procreation. Although many women with disabilities care for small children, the medical system and friends and family often discourage an active sex life and procreation for them, but encourage them for men (Gill 1994).[7] As a result, intimate partnerships between men with disabilities and able-bodied women are more prevalent than between women with disabilities and able-bodied men (Bullard and Knight 1981).

Conventional gender norms permeate sexual behavior, and social constructions of sexuality magnify the effects of physiological disabilities on sexual functioning.[8] Robert Murphy, a paraplegic, recognizes the variety of human sexual practices and pleasures, but he bleakly assesses the situation for paralyzed men:

> Most forms of paraplegia and quadriplegia cause male impotence and female inability to orgasm. But paralytic women need not be aroused or experience orgasmic pleasure to engage in genital sex, and many indulge regularly in intercourse and even bear children, although by Caesarean section. . . . Paraplegic women claim to derive psychological gratification from the sex act itself, as well as from the stimulation of other parts of their bodies and the knowledge that they are still able to give pleasure to others. . . . Males have far more circumscribed anatomical limits. Other than having a surgical implant that produces a simulated erection, the man can no longer engage in genital sex. He either becomes celibate or practices oral sex—or any of the many other variations in sexual expression devised by our innovative species. Whatever the alternative, his standing as a man has been compromised far more than has been the woman's status. He has been effectively emasculated. (1990, 96)

In contrast, Irving Kenneth Zola, whose legs were wasted from polio, described mutual love-making with a severely paralyzed woman, an activity that began with his doing all her physical care, as well as the more conventional undressing, but nonetheless feeling that she had made love to him as well:

> And so the hours passed, ears, mouths, eyes, tongues inside one another. And every once in a while she would quiver in a way which seemed orgasmic. As I thrust my tongue as deep as I could in her ear, her head would begin to shake, her neck would stretch out and then her whole upper body would release with a sigh. . . . So we . . . hugged and curled up as closely

as we could, with my head cradled in her arm and my leg draped across her. . . . I fell quickly asleep— . . . rested, cared for, and loved. (1982b, 216)

The difference in these two versions of sexuality lies in how love-making is defined—whether the physiological or emotional aspects are emphasized and whether sex is defined only as penile penetration. In Murphy's definition of male sexuality, a man who could not use his penis in intercourse is not really a man; Zola's definition of sexuality is not only more egalitarian, its diffuseness encourages many forms of manhood—and womanhood. Those women and men with disabilities who are sexually experimental are more likely to have heterosexual and homosexual partners. Since women seem to be able to achieve orgasm through diffuse sexual excitement and men tend to focus their sexual behavior genitally, women with disabilities may have an advantage in that they are more willing to engage in a variety of sexual practices.

In other respects, they are disadvantaged. For women and men of any sexual orientation who have disabilities, social life is complicated not only by physiological differences that hamper conventional forms of sexual activity, but by difficulties in dating, going to parties, and casual socializing (Clare 1999). One lesbian who lost her eyesight long after she came out writes of missing terribly "regular validation of my status through visual interaction with other dykes"—the winks and smiles exchanged with strangers who recognize they are members of the same community (Peifer 1999, 33). She has the dislocating sense of living in two disparate worlds. A lesbian mother with no hearing feels that she and her nonhearing school-age daughter live in communities that have little overlap and, sometimes, little tolerance of diversity (D'aoust 1999). These communities are the world of the physically challenged (she uses a wheelchair for mobility), the deaf, White mothers of adopted non-White children, and lesbians. She says of her daughter that she "is part of a community that welcomes Deaf people as members but does not have the same history of dealing with other differences" (p. 117).

The problems of women with disabilities are frequently not physical but social—dating and being thought of in a sexual rather than platonic manner, especially during adolescence (Rousso 1988). They are likely to be stigmatized as potential sexual partners even when their disabilities are sensory—blindness and deafness (Becker and Jauregui 1985; Kolb 1985). Women with disabilities tend to have the same sexual attitudes and desires as able-bodied women, but they are less likely to find heterosexual partners than men with disabilities (DeHaan and Wallander 1988). As for homosexual relationships, Rousso (1988) reports that lesbianism and bisexuality occurred among women with disabilities later in life, and without a period of adolescent sexual exploration.

When they do have sexual relationships, women with disabilities find it difficult to obtain contraception or gynecological care commensurate with their physical needs, and their desire to have children is ignored or discounted (Killoran 1994; Waxman 1994). Sexual relations and fatherhood are considered normal aspirations for men with physical disabilities, but women with physical disabilities are often treated like asexual children. Carol Gill says that even after the passage of the Americans with Disabilities Act, "I am treated as though I don't belong with the other women who seek services in OB/GYN unless I can make my disability issues go away" (1994, 117). Interviews with thirty-one women with a variety of disabilities, ranging in age from twenty-two to sixty-nine, well-educated and highly productive, and of different racial ethnic groups, revealed "the common experience of having their reproductive needs undervalued. Many said their physicians treated them as asexual, thought they should not be having children, and assumed that they would not be having children and that they did not want menstrual periods. In many cases, the first recommendation offered was to have a hysterectomy" (Nosek et al. 1995, 512).

Zola comments that "our society does not like to picture people who are weak, sick, and even dying, having needs for sexual intimacy" (1982a, 214). He found that there were few apartments for couples in an otherwise comprehensive living facility in the Netherlands, and that a Swedish project that encouraged the sexual involvement of able-bodied counselors with people with severe disabilities was discontinued because the counselors "actually began to find these very physically disabled people attractive, and *that* was regarded as shocking if not sick" (p. 215).

A recognition of the sexuality of women and men with long-term physiological problems would go a long way toward eroding the stereotypes of both gender and disability. Such rethinking involves breaking down the conventional categorization of women with disabilities as asexual and childlike and men with disabilities as severely frustrated in their sexual expression. In a more general sense, the same depolarization of men versus women and disabled versus able-bodied is necessary to change the social status of those with long-term physiological problems from "outsider" to "one of us."

Toward a Continuum of Bodiedness

One feminist view of women with disabilities argues that they are "doubly handicapped"—by their gender and by their physical limitations (Deegan and Brooks 1985; Morris 1993). In this view, a physical disability is a "minority" status added to all the other jeopardies suffered (Deegan 1985). This view does not address the complexity of intertwined statuses— the status dilemma when a highly placed person becomes disabled or the synergistic effect of a multitude of disadvantages.

Minority-group status allows for activism and fighting for civil rights on the basis of shared interests that enlist people with very different needs. The disability rights movement in the United States successfully fought for ramps in all public buildings, wheelchair-accessible bathrooms, wheelchair lifts in buses, apartments equipped for independent living, braille numbers and bells to indicate floor stops in elevators, closed-captioned television programs, infra-red hearing devices in theaters, sign-language translation at public forums, telephone devices and communications relays, and so on. The movement has also produced antidiscrimination legislation for jobs and housing in pursuit of the goal to integrate people with disabilities into mainstream life.

However, just as feminism has been accused of not attending to the multiple disadvantages of women of color, a broad-based disability rights movement does not address gender differences any more than it does racial or sexual differences that compound discriminatory treatment (Wendell 1992). The goal of the disability-rights movement is to find alternative ways to accomplish the tasks of daily living, ways that may be different for women and men when their family situations are different. When their goals are the same—to hold down a paying job, for example—women with disabilities may need more of what women in general need to counter both sexism and prejudice against those with physical impairments. A determined effort at inclusion of people of different genders, racial ethnic identities, parental status, and sexual orientation, as well as different ranges of bodily capabilities, is more effective here than tackling one problem at a time.

Just as the integration of people with disabilities into the mainstream of society depends on attention to their bodily needs by environmental modifications, access to technology, and personal care attendants, the special biological needs of women with disabilities cannot be ignored. Menstruation, contraception, pregnancy, and childbirth are not problems to be done away with by early hysterectomies, but challenges to health professionals. The extensive repertoire of technologies to assist procreation in women (and men) with infertility problems should certainly be available to those with other disabilities as well. Despite evidence that a woman with disabilities can run households, take care of children, and also work outside the home, the perception still persists that these tasks are impossible for her (Killoran 1994; Shaul et al. 1985). Women with quite severe physical limitations have devised ways of caring for small children: "One mother who could not use her arms found that her two children both learned to scramble up her and hang around her neck" (Lonsdale 1990, 79). Carrie Killoran says of her own parenting, "People with disabilities are already accustomed to doing everything differently and more slowly, and caring for children is no different" (1994, 122; also see Kocher 1994).

The conventional norms of femininity have locked women with disabilities into a paradoxical situation—as women, it is all right for them to be helpless and dependent, but, because they are disabled, they are unlikely to have a man to take care of them. Feminists have argued that norms of independence and economic self-support provide a better model for all women, and that giving women with disabilities the means to accomplish these goals would go a long way toward enhancing their self-esteem and quality of life (Asch and Fine 1988). For men with disabilities, the change has to come in challenges to conventional masculinity. Men could expand their options by having different kinds of relationships rather than overburdening one caregiving woman. Both women and men might welcome group living, but it would have to be autonomous and without restrictions on sexual coupling and children.

Gender expectations and assumptions are harder to change than the physical environment and job requirements. If social groups parcel out roles on the basis of gender, then identity as a woman and a man are tied to being able to fulfill these gender-appropriate roles. Looking at the problem of masculinity and physical disability in the lives of ten men, Thomas Gerschick and Adam Stephen Miller (1994) discovered three strategies: reliance on conventional norms and expectations of manhood, reformulation of these norms, and creation of new norms. The men who relied on the predominant ideals of masculinity felt they had to demonstrate physical strength, athleticism, sexual prowess, and independence. Their self-image was tied into heroics and risk-taking, but they often felt inadequate and incomplete because they couldn't do what they wanted or go where they wanted. The men who reformulated these norms defined their ways of coping with their physical limitations as demonstrations of strength and independence. For example, two quadriplegics who needed round-the-clock personal care assistants did not feel they were dependent on others, but had hired helpers whom they directed and controlled. The men who rejected the standard version of masculinity put more emphasis on relationships than on individual accomplishments, were comfortable with varieties of sexuality, and felt they were nonconformists.

To erase the status dilemmas of women and men with physical disabilities, conventional norms about bodies, functions, beauty, and sexuality need to be reexamined (Asch and Fine 1988; Wendell 1996). Making the experiences of women and people of color visible forced a reconsideration of stereotypes of normality and otherness; similarly, because "physically disabled people have experiences which are not available to the able-bodied, they are in a better position to transcend cultural mythologies about the body" (Wendell 1992, 77). Few people are as beautiful as movie stars or as muscular as body builders. A woman without arms or legs claimed the statue of Venus de Milo as her model of beauty (Frank 1988). Orgasms can be felt in many parts of the body other than the genitals. Races can be run in wheelchairs as well as on foot, on horses, on bicycles, and in cars.

Bodies matter to the person with pain, limited mobility, and sensory difficulties, but the way they matter is also a social phenomenon (Butler 1993; Wendell 1996). One answer to the status contradictions imposed on people with disabilities is to discard the concept of "other." A study of nondisabled people who had long-term relationships with people with extremely severe disabilities found that the "partnership" was based on a sense of essential humanity and full integration into each other's social space (Bogdan and Taylor 1989). Ability and disability, bodily integrity and bodily dysfunction, standards of beauty are all relative, for women and for men. The variety of bodies and social environments make all of us part of a complex continuum of able-bodiness, just as the variety of women and men calls into question gender stereotypes. As Susan Wendell says:

> We need to integrate the experience and knowledge of people with disabilities and those who are dying into the mainstream of our cultures, into our concept of life as it is ordinarily lived. We need to learn to accept that people are not always able to control their bodies and to stop holding them responsible for doing the impossible. In short, we need to become more willing to face the realities of bodily life. (Wendell 1996, 111)

Everyone cannot maintain the same level of physical exertion at all times. Even common conditions—such as cardiac or breathing problems,

difficulty with walking, advanced pregnancy—often need to be compensated for. Yet people with disabilities are not seen as part of a continuum
but as qualitatively different. People who are seen as qualitatively different are often stigmatized. Stigma depends more on what can be seen than
on what can be done: "The person who looks relatively 'normal' but is severely limited by what she can do yields a different cultural figure from
the person who performs life activities successfully—often with aids—but
who looks 'abnormal.'" (Thomson 1994, 590).[9] Women and men with disabilities are praised for the heroic ways in which they live "normal" lives,
but there is always an undercurrent of "difference."

Summary

Women and men whose disabilities allow similar levels of physical functioning have very different life chances. Women are less likely to find jobs
that allow them to be economically independent and are more disadvantaged socially than men with disabilities. If they are heterosexual, they are
less likely to have a lifetime partner, because they need the care and attention that women are expected to give to others, whereas men with
disabilities are more likely to find a life partner. Although many women
with disabilities fill all the domestic responsibilities of wives and are excellent mothers, gender stereotypes often do not give them a chance to take
on those roles. In contrast, as long as a man can be income-producing, he
can fulfill the traditional husband role.

Severely disabled women and men are not expected to be sexual, or
even have sexual desires, yet given the opportunity, they engage in varied
and mutually satisfying lovemaking. Similarly, the gynecological and procreative aspects of the lives of women with disabilities are minimized or
ignored by the medical community, who often advocate hysterectomies
rather than giving advice about contraception and fertility.

Care and personal assistance, whether by kin or professionals, is another gendered issue. Women kin are expected to be caregivers, even
though men can be as adept and skilled and are usually the professional
personal assistants for men with disabilities. The expectation of altruism
and sacrifice puts the burdens of care on women, so that men are often
deemed "heroic" when they take on these roles for friends or family members. Because of the lack of social preparation, however, men may break
down more severely under the emotional responsibilities.

Bodily ability for everyone is a continuum that changes throughout our lives, and many of us who consider ourselves "able-bodied" are hampered by physical deficiencies and grateful for the environmental and technological easements many countries have mandated for public facilities and workplaces. People with disabilities are part of this continuum, yet they still tend to be isolated and stigmatized as "different." They are as different among themselves—by all the usual social measures, but especially gender—as any other supposedly uniform group of people.

Notes

1. This chapter does not discuss emotional or learning disabilities; they are beyond the focus of this book.

2. "Disabilities Affect One-Fifth of Americans." Census Brief, 1997, U.S. Census Bureau Web site.

3. People with *status dilemmas* have two contradictory major statuses, one high and one low (Hughes 1971).

4. For accounts of lesbians with disabilities, see Brownworth and Raffo (1999).

5. For a poignant, detailed account by a man of his care of his wife in the last stages of Alzheimer's, see Bayley (1998).

6. I am indebted to Susan Farrell for this point.

7. See the special issue of *Sexuality and Disability* 12 (Summer): 1994, "Women with Disabilities: Reproduction and Motherhood," edited by Marsha Saxton.

8. For personal testimonies and counseling advice on these issues, see Bullard and Knight (1981).

9. An Israeli study found that parents were more likely to reject a newborn with what they felt were "non-human" facial or bodily deformities that were non-life-threatening than one with serious, but hidden, defects (Weiss 1994).

CHAPTER 5

If a Situation Is Defined as Real: Premenstrual Syndrome and Menopause

We should think about the consequences of defining a large proportion of otherwise well women as ill because of unpleasant feelings during part of their menstrual cycle. To assert the reality of their feelings—yes, this is essential—but to decide that they are abnormal and to be stamped out . . . that is another matter. (Laws et al. 1985, 36)

In the twentieth century, in Western culture, the menstrual cycle was transformed from a misunderstood and somewhat contaminating female phenomenon to a series of biomedical events—the hormonal inputs of puberty, preparation of the uterus for pregnancy, and cessation of reproductive function. From this biologically informed perspective, we learn that for most women, in the absence of conception, menstruation ensues; if a heterosexually active teenage to middle-aged woman doesn't get her monthly period, she suspects that she is pregnant. When a woman's ovaries stop their maturation of eggs, the cessation of ovulation sets off the process we call menopause. A woman's body no longer secretes pregnancy-preparing hormones that thicken the lining of her uterus; the lining no longer needs to be sloughed off in the absence of fertilization of the ovum, and gradually, the cessation of menstrual periods—menopause—occurs.[1] Any problems that accompany these cycles, such as pain, discomfort, or emotional reactions, have become medical. The solution is frequently a prescription for a hormone or other powerful medication, when stress management, nutritional supplements, and social supports might work better and have fewer long-term side effects.

Women's experiences of menarche, menstruation, and menopause are mediated by beliefs about femininity, desirability, and social worth. In Western culture, menarche is not a time of celebration, but the onset of the possible embarrassment of showing blood and the danger of getting pregnant. Menstruation is an occasion for put-downs about poor functioning "on the rag." Menopause has become a sign of aging and the end of procreative capabilities. Since a Western woman's social status is so intertwined with her body and reproductive biology, cultural values surrounding menstruation and menopause spill over into valuations of womanhood itself.

These negative feelings about oneself and one's body can intensify reactions to the cramps, bloating, and other physical reactions that often accompany hormonal fluctuations. Serious attention to these discomforts legitimizes a physical and social reality that historically was ignored, trivialized, or misunderstood. However, the medical and cultural interpretation of these reactions can also stigmatize women as mentally ill, unreliable, sick, incompetent, and weak. Although there certainly are women who do benefit from amelioration of disabling menstrual conditions, most women pursue their usual activities before and during menstruation and menopause (Yankauskas 1990). Nonetheless, there are multiple examples of how all women are said to suffer (and make others suffer in turn) from the "horrors" of "that time of month" or "that time of life." In our society, these syndromes denigrate women as a group and justify their subordinate social status (Laws 1983; Rittenhouse 1991; Zita 1988). Menstruation and menopause are real physiological and emotional events. A gendered analysis of sociocultural and biomedical interpretations of female procreative cycles as the sources of physiological and emotional disorders shows the power and legitimacy of Western medicine to shape these experiences. The onset and cessation of menstruation are now believed to be liminally dangerous times for all women, and this social reality affects women's everyday lives. To paraphrase a classic statement of sociology, "If a situation is defined as real, it is real in its consequences."[2]

Medicalized Menstruation

The events of the menstrual cycle vary in when they occur, how long they are experienced, and what physiological and psychological changes accompany them. In the course of biomedical research on the physiology of the female reproductive system, "normal" was defined and specified: time of first period (menarche), length of time between cycles, duration and amount of flow, timing of cessation of cycles, and physiological and emotional accompaniments to all of these events.[3] The 28-day cycle, which Johanna Foster says is a widely accepted myth in Western culture, is based on an equally conventional month of four seven-day weeks, not on a lunar month, which takes 29.5 days (1996, 536–37). Even the dosage of the oral contraceptives that were so popular in the 1960s and 1970s was geared to a supposed "natural" menstrual cycle (Gladwell 2000). Yet, at present, in medical and popular publications, the divisions of the cycle differ in number, transition points, markers, and names:

> Not only are there discrepancies over how many phases constitute "the menstrual cycle" and what to call these supposedly distinct phases, but there is also contention in the literatures over how long some of these stages should last, particularly "ovulation," "postovulation," "premenstruation," "menstruation," and perhaps most importantly, the whole "menstrual cycle." (Foster 1996, 535)

The biomedical perspective on the physical, behavioral, and emotional effects of the menstrual cycle is thus a social construction, reflecting the high value Western science puts on regularity and control of bodily functions. As Joan Brumberg's (1997) social and cultural history of female bodies demonstrates, the biomedical perspective on menstruation colludes with corporate forces to create a commercial ritual for adolescent girls. Using girls' diaries and media advertisements to investigate the historically changing meaning of menstruation, Brumberg concludes:

> Unfortunately, many American girls grow up equating the experience of menarche and menstruation with a hygiene product. By creating a profit-making enterprise from adolescent self-consciousness, the postwar sanitary products industry paved the way for the commercialization of other areas of the body, such as skin, hair, breasts—all of great concern to developing girls. (p. 54)

Articles on menstrual problems in women's magazines are written by doctors or cite doctors, and the accounts of women's experiences in them reflect the biomedical view that these problems are individual abnormalities caused by imbalanced hormones (Chrisler and Levy 1990; Markens 1996). A medical consultation may or may not help an individual woman with her problem, but it is likely to result in a medical label for her symptoms. From a social perspective, the encouragement of girls and women to seek medical help for any and all menstrual problems contaminates the status of womanhood with the expectation of regularly recurring illness (Riessman 1998). These "illnesses" are various: too frequent or infrequent menstrual periods, premenstrual physical and emotional reactions; difficulties during menstruation—in short, whatever does not meet the current medical measures for normal female functioning.

As a result, women's bodies are routinely made publicly visible, managed, and "protected" by a powerful institution of social control. One consequence is that despite the strong evidence of women's overall physical hardiness, *all* women are considered unfit for certain kinds of work and physical activity because of their procreative physiology. What supposedly makes females "real" women—their menstrual cycles—makes them unreliable workers, thinkers, and leaders.

Cultural Constructions of Menstruation

In many Western folklores, menstruating women are impure and contaminating. In the shift to a scientific view of menstruation in the late nineteenth century, notions of menstrual pollution were replaced by the idea that monthly periods were necessary to women's health (Bullough and Voght 1973). A twentieth-century version that challenges the cultural view that menstruating women are impure transfers the notion of impurity to men. In 1993, in a long article in *The Quarterly Review of Biology*, Margie Profet, a feminist biologist, presented an innovative biological theory of why women menstruate. Profet argued that "the function of menstruation is to defend against pathogens transported to the uterus by sperm" (p. 338). Using data from research on the menstrual cycles of primates and other animals where fertilization is internal, she claimed that the design of the uterus and the non-clotting quality of menstrual blood are evidence of menstruation's protective function in ridding the uterus of potentially harmful bacteria. Thus, in her interpretation, menstruation rids women of impurities instead of making them impure.

In actuality, menstruating is the mark of a woman's potential fertility, and it is her child-bearing capacity that was seen in need of protection, not her health. Thus, when more women began to attend college at the beginning of the twentieth century, scientific studies supposedly proved that if they used their heads too much, they would stop menstruating—they would no longer be fertile women. There were also dire warnings that too much exercise was bad for women's fertility (Vertinsky 1990).

In the late 1970s, as women increasingly entered athletic competitions, similar scientific studies showed that women who exercised intensely would cease menstruating because they would not have enough body fat to sustain ovulation (Brozan 1978). But when one set of researchers did a year-long study that compared 66 women—21 who were training for a marathon, 22 who ran more than an hour a week, and 23 who did less than an hour of aerobic exercise a week—they discovered that only 20 percent of the women in any of these groups had "normal" menstrual cycles every month (Prior et al. 1990). The dangers of intensive training for women's fertility were exaggerated as women began to compete in arenas formerly closed to them.

Emily Martin attributes the proliferation of research on the monthly inefficiency and unreliability of women workers to the goal of keeping them out of the work force during times of high unemployment, such as during the Depression (1992, 113–28). When women workers were necessary to arms production during World War II, other studies (sometimes by the same researchers) showed that menstruation was no hindrance to women doing any kind of work.

According to many feminists, the subordinate social status of women is the result of historic and economic processes; biology is used as a pervasive justification for their subordination but is not the cause of it (Koeske 1983; Lorber 1993b).[4] Gloria Steinem asked in 1978, "What would happen . . . if suddenly, magically, men could menstruate and women could not? . . . The answer is clear—menstruation would become an enviable, boast-worthy, masculine event" (p. 110).

Ritual Menstruation

Non-Western cultural models often present a more positive view of menstruation, construing its phases as positive life cycle events to be ritually celebrated (Buckley and Gottlieb 1988). Chris Knight (1991) has developed a theory that links menstruation and the origin of culture in prehistoric gathering and hunting societies. Using Martha McClintock's (1971) observations that women who live together often menstruate at the same time, Knight argues that since the women of a tribe worked together, they would ovulate and menstruate together.[5] They would then refuse to have sex with the men of the tribe and would encourage them to go away from the camp to hunt. They would induce the men to bring back the meat to be cooked with the promise of sexual relations during what would then be the women's time of greatest fertility. The symbolic taboos on menstrual blood and on the blood of raw meat were, Knight argued, the origins of culture.

The more common conceptualization of menstrual taboos has been negative and oppressive of women: "Perhaps one reason the negative image of failed production is attached to menstruation is precisely that women are in some sinister sense out of control when they menstruate. They are not reproducing, not continuing the species, not preparing to stay at home with the baby, not providing a safe, warm womb to nurture a man's sperm" (Martin 1992, 47).

However, in nonindustrialized societies with high fertility rates, menstruation does not occur every month, since women are pregnant or breast-feeding during most of their child-bearing years. Menstruation is unusual, an anomaly, and it is sometimes seen as conferring magical powers; menstrual blood can be used for witchcraft—to harm or to heal (Buckley and Gottlieb 1988). Close readings of ethnographic accounts reveal that it is often unclear whether menstruating women have to be kept in seclusion because they are contaminating, or others have to be kept away from menstruating women because they are sacred and frightening:

> Many menstrual taboos, rather than protecting society from a universally ascribed feminine evil, explicitly protect the perceived creative spirituality of menstruous women from the influence of others in a more neutral state, as well as protecting the latter in turn from the potent, positive spiritual force ascribed to such women. In other cultures menstrual customs, rather than subordinating women to men fearful of them, provide women with means of ensuring their own autonomy, influence, and social control. (Buckley and Gottlieb 1988, 7)

Whether menstruation stigmatizes or endows women with charisma, it has been seen as something that disturbs the usual social order and must be contained (Martin 1992, 27–53).

Emotional Menstruation

The ideology that women are out of control around the time of menstruation has become attached to the premenstrual syndrome (PMS). Women who experience PMS are said to be particularly excitable during the week or so before they menstruate—exhibiting mood swings, aggressiveness, anger, and even violence. The same notion of uncontrollability colors menopause, the time of cessation of regular menstrual cycles. Here, however, the woman is said to suffer more than those around her—from the embarrassment of hot flashes, insomnia from night sweats, and general emotionality. The onset, occurrence, and cessation of menstruation are caused by hormonal shifts that are, in themselves, normal physiological events that can have diverse bodily and behavioral effects (Lennane and Lennane 1973). The question is, why are these accompanying effects considered "symptoms"? And is the translation of diffuse "feelings" into a clear "diagnosis" benign or detrimental? The answer to the first question depends on a woman's culture and the extent to which the menstrual cycle is medicalized in her social world. The answer to the second question depends on how diagnoses of PMS and menopause are viewed, in medical as well as lay discourse.

The current view of PMS and menopause as producing uncontrollable emotions and behavior is reminiscent of the view of pollution as that which disturbs the social order (Douglas 1966). As Sophie Laws says,

> The "symptoms" of [PMS] which the doctors show most concern over— depression, anxiety, and so on—are mental states which do not "fit" with women's culturally created notions of ourselves as nice, kind, gentle, etc. "Mood change," as such, is often listed as a symptom—demonstrating that change *as such* is not culturally acceptable. . . . There's just no room for women to have strong feelings of their own, disrupting this comfortable flow of emotional services. (Laws et al. 1985, 35)

In this sense, PMS and menopause have replaced menstruation itself as antisocial forces that need to be subdued. To counter this view, some feminists have reinterpreted menstrual mood swings as having positive rather than negative effects, describing, for example, premenstrual tension as a heightened energy state (Guinan 1988).

PMS: Hormonal Hurricane or High Energy State?[6]

Premenstrual tension was described and attributed to hormonal causes sixty-five years ago (Frank 1931); since then, most research has followed the biomedical model—defining it as *a* syndrome, with *a* hormonal cause, *a* pathology located in the *individual*. Much of the medical and lay focus has been on the psychological aspects of what was called Late Luteal Phase Dysphoric Disorder and Premenstrual Dysphoric Disorder in the American Psychiatric Association's official diagnostic manuals (Figert 1995; Gitlin and Pasnau 1989). More recently, the pharmaceutical industry, through a multimedia advertising campaign, has claimed that Premenstrual Dyspho-ric Disorder (PMDD) is a more severe but widely experienced form of PMS. It is cited as an official psychiatric diagnosis with accompanying pharma-ceutical treatments. According to one study done under pharmaceutical auspices, PMDD affects approximately 5 percent of menstruating women in the United States (Frackiewicz and Shiovitz 2001).

Premenstrual psychological effects are genuine problems when they interfere with a woman's capacity to carry on her normal social functions, when they disturb her social relationships, and most notoriously, when they cause violent acting out (Rittenhouse 1991). However, critics have noted that there is considerable confusion about PMS—whether it is a single syn-drome, when it occurs, whether the psychological effects are hormonal, how many women have debilitating effects, and whether the effects are neces-sarily negative.

The diffuseness and multiplicity of symptoms are indications of diag-nostic slipperiness—close to one hundred different symptoms of PMS have been listed (Laws et al. 1985, 37–38). Some women experience premenstrual bodily changes, others emotional ups and downs, and still others a combi-nation of both, in mild, moderate, and severe forms:

> The emotional states most commonly reported in studies of PMS are ten-sion, anxiety, depression, irritability, and hostility. Somatic complaints in-clude abdominal bloating, swelling, breast tenderness, headache, and backache. Behavioral changes frequently reported are an avoidance of so-cial contact, a change in work habits, increased tendency to pick fights (es-pecially with a spouse/partner or children), and crying spells. (Abplanalp 1983, 109)

There is some question about the cyclicity of PMS. Many women and men experience mood swings by the day of the week; for women, these may modify or intensify menstrual-cycle mood swings (Hoffmann 1982; Rossi and Rossi 1977). Mary Brown Parlee (1982b) found that individual women were less likely to attribute psychological mood swings to men-strual cycles than to other causes, such as reactions to difficulties at work or at home; when the data were grouped, however, the presence of men-strual mood cycles was magnified because the other patterns were idiosyncratic. Daily self-reports gave "a picture of what might be called a 'premenstrual elation syndrome' that is the opposite of the negative one embodied in the stereotype of premenstrual tension" (Parlee 1982b, 130). Retrospective reports from these same women described their feelings in stereotypically gendered terms. They interpreted PMS as a medically permissible aberration from otherwise socially expected performances of femininity.

Stereotypically, women suffering from PMS are said to be cranky, irritable, angry, violent, out of control. These characteristics assume some kind of comparison—with the same woman at other times of the month or with an idealized notion of the behavior of a "normal" feminine, heterosexual woman of reproductive age. One woman physician sardonically commented that perhaps the effects of what is defined as premenstrual syndrome—anger and irritability—stand out because this behavior is in contrast to three weeks of pleasant sociability (Guinan 1988). Sharon Golub suggests that comparisons with men would be useful: "While women's moods may vary cyclically, there is no evidence that women are more prone to anger than men. In fact, the opposite is probably true. Witness the far higher rates of crime and accidents among men. Some have suggested that the worst part of being premenstrual is that that is when women are most like men" (Golub 1992, 204).

Control groups, however, are rarely used in research on PMS (Fausto-Sterling 1985, 106–7). Samples are usually not diversified by racial or ethnic group, religion, social class, age, or sexual orientation, nor are cycles followed for a long period of time. Subjective feelings of tension, agitation, depression, and anger are loosely defined and poorly measured. The menstrual cycle is assumed to be the cause of mood changes, never the other way around, even though research has shown that hormones are as affected by behavior as behavior is by hormones (Kemper 1990; Koeske 1983). The notorious connection between premenstrual tension and crimes, suicides, and other destructive actions may be due to emotional stress that causes both changes in the menstrual cycle and pathological behavior. Brown Parlee (1982a) found that women taking important examinations are as likely to be premenstrual or menstruating as women committing crimes are.

The controversy over whether PMS could be used as a defense in murder trials made the syndrome a household word in 1981 (Laws 1983). An equally contentious battle went on during the late 1980s over whether to make PMS an official diagnosis in the revised third edition of the *Diagnostic and Statistical Manual of Mental Disorders* (DSM-III-R), which delayed its publication by two years (Figert 1995). In this battle, the feminist Committee on Women of the American Psychiatric Association (APA) enlisted professional and lay women's groups to prevent the legitimation of a diagnosis that they felt had the potential of stigmatizing all menstruating women as potentially "crazy." They argued that even a careful definition that emphasized severity and intractability of psychological reactions to a primarily physiological phenomenon was likely to be misconstrued as constantly recurring instability and irrationality. However, without an official diagnosis, third-party insurers would not pay for treatment of PMS as a primary psychiatric disorder.

The issue of who was to treat was interwoven with the question of the definition of the disorder (Figert 1995). If the problem is due to hormonal imbalance, then it is the province of gynecologists; if the problem is primarily emotional, then it should be treated by M.D. psychiatrists. Psychologists, social workers, and other mental health workers who did not have M.D. degrees claimed the right to treat what they defined as a social situational problem. Feminist women's groups pushed for self-treatment and alternative health care remedies for the discomforts of a normal physiological process. The Institute for Research on Women's Health in Washington, D.C., using feminist networks and the mailing list of the National Coalition for Women's Mental Health, focused media and the public's attention on the issue, and encouraged a letter-writing campaign to the APA.

The outcome was a compromise—listing in the Appendix of the DSM-III-R and also in the DSM-IV. Such placement indicates that the syndrome needs additional research for verification and use as an insurable diagnosis. It was a defeat for the professional and laywomen who wanted to keep PMS out of the manual entirely, Figert argues, and a victory for the PMS researchers who wanted criteria to make their research "more definable, specific, and fundable" (1995, 68). But the criteria (physical and psychological, not social situational) then shape the way the research is designed and predicts the ultimate outcome (medical or psychological treatment, not changes in relationships or lifestyle). As Brown Parlee points out, the call for more rigorous criteria of menstrual cycles frequently means that even in social scientists' research, physiological measurements of hormonal levels are built into the research design, necessitating collaboration with biomedically trained researchers (1994, 98).

Although positive mood changes have been reported for over a decade, they are almost never looked for in most PMS research (Martin 1992, 128–29; Parlee 1982b). Martin suggests that from a feminist perspective, premenstrual tension can be positive—not only a release of ordinarily suppressed anger at the everyday put-downs women are subject to, but a different kind of consciousness, concentration, and creativity: "Does the loss of ability to concentrate mean a greater ability to free-associate? Loss of muscle control, a gain in ability to relax? Decreased efficiency, increased attention to a smaller number of tasks?" (1992, 128). Women who have autonomy in their work could find these times productive, but factory workers, data processors, nurses, mothers of small children—the majority of women—cannot afford the loss of self-discipline. Given the way work and time are organized in industrialized societies, "women are perceived as malfunctioning and their hormones out of balance rather than the organization of society and work perceived as in need of a transformation to demand less constant discipline and productivity" (Martin 1992, 123). Since work and family life are not likely to be reorganized, women who are overwhelmed by the pressures of their daily lives may find it necessary to claim illness periodically, as a means of getting relief without blame (Parlee 1994, 104–5).

Menopause: The End of Womanhood or the Beginning of a Valued Status?

As with PMS, the biomedical accounts of menopause have outweighed social analysis and commentary in professional and lay discourse (Bell 1990). Western culture imposes a negative connotation on women's experiences of their bodies and emphasizes a separation of body and mind. Western women are given no chance to contemplate their bodies as located in time and place and as *theirs* to control (Levesque-Lopman 1988). Women experience menopause as a culturally constructed process mediated by beliefs about femininity, desirability, and productivity. It has become a sign of aging and the end of procreative capabilities. Since Western women's social status is so intertwined with their body and biology, menopause has been seen as virtually the end of womanhood (Zita 1993). In contrast, Peruvian women gain full adulthood around the time of menopause, reaping social and financial benefits and freedom from daily chores for large extended families (Barnett 1988).

Affluent men or those who have attained secure positions in academe or other professions had, in the past, not worried as much about aging as middle-class women had, but their cultural protections may be disappearing. The highly fluctuating economy and women's growing financial and psychological independence make men vulnerable to the marketing of facelifts and other cosmetic surgery, hair transplants and dyes, exercise and sports regimens (Gullette 1993). Despite talk of a male climacteric, the markers of aging in men are not yet as medicalized as menopause is. So the pressures on men to "do something about aging" are less likely to be backed by a powerful medical ideology that translates natural processes into illness and routinizes hormonal replacement therapy in the name of "feminine forever."[7] No one seems to be arguing that men over fifty are not masculine.

What makes menopause different from PMS is that the condition itself, not just its effects, is seen as a medical problem. Cessation of menstruation, the result of no longer ovulating, has become a "deficiency disease" to be cured by permanent hormone replacement therapy (McCrea 1986). Despite the evidence of lay knowledge about menopause and treatment of its accompanying effects by herbal medicines and high-soy and other diets, biomedical treatments are assumed to be the only legitimate resource (Agee 2000; Goldstein 2000). The use of estrogen, popularized in the 1960s, was supposed to cure psychological as well as physiological effects of menopause—to energize, tranquilize, counteract depression, increase libido, alleviate hot flashes, minimize night sweating, and reverse vaginal dryness. By the mid-1970s, the danger of endometrial cancer led to medical recommendations that estrogen, also known as hormone replacement therapy (HRT), be used only for symptoms directly related to lower hormone levels (body temperature fluctuations and vaginal changes), at low doses, and for a short period of time. Instead, drug companies came up with an estrogen-progesterone combination that they claimed was safer, although there were reports of possible increases the incidence of breast cancer with its long-term use (Lewis 1993).

Around the same time, a new reason for extended use of HRT emerged—preventing the loss of bone mass and forestalling the possible development of osteoporosis. A recent clinical conference on osteoporosis recommended a combination of prevention tactics in addition to HRT—calcium in diet and supplements, exercise to increase bone mass and strengthen muscles, balance training, stopping smoking (Anonymous 2001; see also Cauley et al. 2001). An additional indication for long-term hormone replacement is prevention of heart disease, but HRT use is not unequivocally beneficial (Grodstein et al. 2001; Mosca et al. 2001). Perhaps because of the complexity of treatment outcomes and side effects, many women find it difficult to decide whether to go on or continue long-term hormone use, even though it is heavily promoted by physicians and by the pharmaceutical industry (Griffiths 1999).

Early studies of symptoms of menopause were done on women who had sought medical help or who had had hysterectomies. In order to track the occurrence of perimenopausal, menopausal, and postmenopausal symptoms in a more general population, a cohort of 2,572 women aged forty-five to fifty-five years in 1981 were selected from census lists in thirty-eight Massachusetts cities and towns (Avis and McKinlay 1995).[8] The sample was diversified by size of city or town, per capita income, and racial identification. The women were interviewed for thirty minutes by telephone every nine months over five years. At each interview, they were asked questions about their menstrual status, physical health, utilization of health care, and sociodemographic status. On a rotating basis, they were asked about their social support networks, their lifestyle (including depression), and their help-seeking behavior. This carefully constructed survey found that "natural menopause seems to have no major impact on health or health behavior. The majority of women do not seek additional help concerning menopause, and their attitudes toward it are, overwhelmingly, positive or neutral" (Avis and McKinlay 1995, 45). Almost 69 percent of the women did not report being bothered by hot flashes or night sweats, and 23 percent did not report having had them at all. Only 32 percent said they had consulted a doctor for menopausal-related symptoms, and these women were likely to have been depressed before menopause. The authors conclude that the stressful impact of other life events far outweighs the stress of menopause.

Other studies have also shown that the incidence of supposedly universal symptoms of menopause are not experienced by every woman. Japanese women are much less likely to report experiencing hot flashes or night sweats during the year after their menses had ceased than women in Manitoba, Canada, and Massachusetts in the United States (Lock 1993, 36).[9] Interviews with 603 postmenopausal Indonesian women found that less than a third reported having had hot flashes; they used an herbal drink and daily servings of papaya (which is estrogenic) as a remedy for hot flashes and for vaginal dryness (Flint and Samil 1990). A Netherlands study of 4,426 women and 4,253 men between the ages of twenty-five and seventy-five used data from a general health questionnaire administered to a sample of general practitioners' patients (Van Hall et al. 1994). The researchers found that the only symptom directly related to menopause was excessive perspiration. Diffuse complaints, such as dizziness, headache, tiredness, nervousness, sleeplessness, listlessness, palpitations, aggressivity, irritability, and depression were neither gender-specific nor age-specific. These authors concluded that "there is no rationale in prescribing estrogens for psychological problems or mood disorders occurring during the climacteric or the postmenopausal period" (p. 47).

Margaret Lock's study of menopause in Japan found that it was not medicalized: "The dominant physicians' discourse, which they share with nearly all their patients, remains one in which *konenki* figures as a natural transition, one through which both men and women must pass, but during which, because of their biological makeup, women are thought to be more vulnerable than men to physical and emotional difficulties" (1993, 293). A visit to a physician is encouraged for women only to check that there are no other health problems, and hormonal replacement therapy is used very conservatively; herbal medicine is preferred. Without widespread use of hormonal replacement, Japanese women have one-quarter the mortality rate from heart disease and half the incidence of osteoporosis of North American Caucasian women, despite a less dense bone mass; their life expectancy is the longest in the world (pp. 295–96).

Menopausal symptoms are not even universal among inhabitants of the same country. As part of the Study of Women's Health Across the Nation (SWAN), researchers interviewed 14,906 multiethnic, multiracial, middle-aged women. Based on self-reported medical histories from women of Caucasian, African-American, Chinese, Japanese, and Hispanic groups, the consistently statistically significant factors that were identified as experienced during menopause were hot flashes and night sweats (vasomotor symptoms) and psychological and psychosomatic symptoms, such as depression and headaches (Avis et al. 2001). Controlling for age, education, health, and economic status, Caucasian women reported significantly more psychological symptoms and African-American women reported significantly more vasomotor symptoms. The variety of ways menopause is experienced by different women has been termed "local biologies," suggesting that there is no universal menopausal "syndrome" (Lock and Kaufert 2001).

If menstruating is so problematic, why is the cessation of menstruation construed as such a problem, asks Sharon Golub, and gives as the answer, "fear: fear of aging, fear of loss of sexuality, fear of getting depressed, fear of loss of health" (1992, 236). Yet when these connotations of menopause are teased apart, the health aspect elicits more negative attitudes than when menopause is construed as a sign of aging, like gray hair and retirement, or when it is seen as a life transition, like puberty and leaving home (Gannon and Ekstrom 1993). Furthermore, women on the other side of the menstrual divide, those who are a year past their last period, have expressed very positive feelings—"of beginning a new life, of feeling great, of being wonderful, and of enjoying their lives" (Dickson 1990). The study of postmenopausal Indonesian women also found a high incidence of reports of positive feelings—affection, excitement, well-being, energy, and orderliness (Flint and Samil 1990).

Feminist analyses look beyond the individual to sociocultural phenomena—the social status of older women, differing images of sexuality for women and men, and place in a constellation of family and friends.[10] These phenomena, which vary from culture to culture and by social class, structure the experience of menopause. Thus, aging women in the United States are supposed to turn to their doctors for help; in Japan, they expect to be looked after by their daughters-in-law (Lock 1993, 386). Among upper-caste women in India who are segregated from men, menopause lifts their restrictions and gives them the freedom to socialize outside the home and to travel (Flint 1982, 367–69). For American women, "it meant pleasure at avoiding whatever discomfort they felt during periods and relief from the nuisance of dealing with bleeding, pads, or tampons. . . . For those women sexually active with men, it meant delight to not suffer the fear of pregnancy" (Martin 1982, 175). But not an elevation to a more valued status.

Marcha Flint's suggestion for Western women is to "bring all aged crones into view, not as spectral shadows, but as women in our full presence, substance, and power" (1993, 75). Germaine Greer's manifesto is even more confrontational: "Though the old woman is both feared and reviled, she need not take the intolerance of others to heart, for women over fifty already form one of the largest groups in the population structure of the Western world" (1991, 4).

Politics of PMS and Menopause

Reviewing her own twenty years of work on menstruation, the conferences she has attended, and the proliferating literature on PMS, Mary Brown Parlee concludes that "biomedical researchers' knowledge claims . . . have come to prevail over those of social scientists. . . . As in the popular culture, biomedical literature now routinely and unproblematically (incontestably) refers to PMS as some*thing* some women 'have.' Permitted scientific disputes now concern what causes 'it' and how 'it' can be treated" (1994, 103). The same thing, she suggests, has happened to menopause. In both instances, drug companies profit from enormous markets for their products; gynecologists profit from expansion of their practices in a time of declining births; psychiatrists (especially those in managed care) also benefit from a larger pool of patients; physician-researchers' quantifiable projects get funds from government agencies, medical centers, and drug companies. A longitudinal study found an overall trend of increases in estrogen prescriptions from 1980 to 1995, indicating the predominance of the medical system in defining and treating menopause (Bartman and Moy 1998).

However, it is not simply entrepreneurial interests that drive the trend of medicalizing women's bodies and procreative experiences. In the medicalization of PMS and menopause, one of the main interest groups has been women themselves. The biomedical model of PMS and menopause has advantages for women. Just as in the late nineteenth century, when middle- and upper-class women used the sick role as a way of opting out of the obligation to bear numerous children and run households to suit their husband's wishes, women today may get temporary relief from multitasking and a partner's attention to their needs with a diagnosis of menstrual complications legitimated by the ultimate authority, the physician (Ehrenreich and English 1973; Parlee 1994). For working-class women with access to medical care, who had no such recourse in the nineteenth century, medical attention may be better than no attention.

When PMS and menopause produce debilitating physical and psychological symptoms for certain women, prescriptions for tranquilizers, mood enhancers, and hormone replacement have certainly been helpful. But so have herbal remedies, dietary supplements, exercise, and yoga. So, what are the dangers of the medical diagnosis of PMS and menopause? First, it frequently results in treatments that have bad side effects. Second, it objectifies and pathologizes women's bodies and procreative cycles. Third, it focuses attention only on the negative aspects, the concomitant discomforts and emotional upsets that bring a woman to the doctor, and ignores the positive aspects frequently reported in field surveys. Fourth, it makes women periodically "sick," and their reputations as reliable workers, and especially their potential for positions of authority, are seriously damaged. And finally, women's anger and protest over the conditions of their lives are safely defused by a diagnosis that can be contained within the medical system.

Transforming Diagnoses Back into Women's Troubles

Since so much of the current perspective on PMS and menopause is bio-medical, it is important to look at what goes on in the doctor's office that turns presenting symptoms into medical diagnoses. In her analysis of medical encounters between women patients and men doctors, Kathy Davis describes how patients' emotionally loaded reports of diffuse complaints are shaped and focused into treatable medical syndromes by doctors who are genuinely trying to ameliorate the patients' distress (1988, 330–46). Her accounts suggest the process by which women's search for help for disturbances of the body and emotions around the times of menstruation and its cessation get turned into medical diagnoses.

In presenting their reasons for coming to the doctor, Davis notes, patients not only describe their symptoms or the progress of an ongoing illness, they also complain about their social troubles, their suffering, their distress: "Patients defined their problems as part of the activity of complaining rather than as a complaint, as an experience rather than a diagnostic category, as something serious enough to feel bad about, and themselves as persons deserving both sympathy and respect" (p. 333). The physicians' task is to use medical expertise to sort out what is significant in the patient's "story about trouble." The physician could tell the patient that she had no treatable medical condition and just listen for the time allotted for the visit. But physicians are trained to "do something," and so they adapt the patient's presenting complaints to fit the most likely medical diagnosis and urge the patient to accept it and the treatment that goes with it.

The encounter, Davis notes, is not one of overt power and coercion. The patient comes to the doctor as an expert for help with something she feels she cannot handle on her own. The doctor, in turn, feels obligated to offer practical help. Since the physician's perspective and knowledge are biomedical, the patient's troubles are transformed into a medical diagnosis. What is medically significant is the patient's physiological or psychosomatic reactions, and not the patient's social situation or social status. The remedy is a prescription for medication, not help in understanding what is wrong in the patient's life or support for doing something about her troubles herself. "Not only were the women's problems shorn of their contextuality and forced into professional schemes of relevance, but the GP seemed unable, in many cases, to understand what made the problems problematic in the first place" (p. 345).

Although Davis did not have a comparison group of women physicians, Sue Fisher's (1995) work on the similarities and differences of women patients' medical encounters with men physicians and women nurse-practitioners suggests that even health care workers committed to a caring style maintain asymmetrical power, set the limits of appropriate topics for discussion, and pressure for compliance with what they think is the best treatment. The nurse-practitioners do, however, pay much more attention to the patient's accounts of their lifestyles and current social situations, grant more competence and knowledge to their patients as women, and are less likely to reproduce conventional ideas about appropriate feminine roles and behavior. They also tend to suggest treatments tailored to a patient's specific needs.

Women physicians are located between men physicians and women nurse-practitioners in the medical hierarchy. Unless they have set up a consciously feminist and patient-oriented practice, they may not act differently than men toward women patients (Lorber 1985). However, as we saw from the research on the medical encounter, women physicians do listen and talk more. They are as likely as men physicians, though, to use medical diagnoses of menopausal problems and suggest treatment by drugs or hormones (Bush 1992).

It is probable that only by going outside of the conventional medical system can menstrual and menopausal discomforts be demedicalized. Alternative healing practices, such as diet, massage, exercise, and nutritional and herbal remedies, may be more appropriate to the diffuse and periodic symptoms so embedded in a woman's daily life than the hormones and tranquilizers doctors are likely to prescribe (Harrison 1985).[11] But the search for treatment does not resolve the larger question of why the subtle or marked physical and emotional changes that accompany menstrual cycles are considered abnormal and social problems and not part of normal variations in the rhythm of days, weeks, months, and years. For that, a different perspective is needed, one that is fully aware of gender issues, as well as the accompanying effects of racial ethnic discrimination, social class inequities, relationship status, parental responsibilities, work pressures, and all the other situational aspects of women's whole lives:

> If we are to respect ourselves as women we have to own all our states of being as parts of ourselves, even, and perhaps especially, the painful ones. If we are angry or sad before our periods, there is anger or sadness in us, and there are reasons for it. The menstrual cycle does not impose extraneous problems on a woman—it is part of her. (Laws et al. 1985, 57–58)

Summary

In this chapter we have argued that a biomedical focus on menstruation and the menopause, currently the perspective legitimated by medicine and scientific research, can have dangerous consequences for individual women and for the status of women in Western society. Medical attention turns diffuse physiological and psychological symptoms into diagnoses of illness. Reports in the scientific and lay media ignore positive feelings frequently reported in surveys and interviews of women who do not consult doctors—feelings of elation, energy, and well-being.

While the treatment of premenstrual, menstrual, and menopausal physiological and psychological effects do bring relief to women who suffer from them, the syndromes have been stretched into expectable stages of every woman's life. These syndromes then contaminate the social status of women in general because they are cited as validations of women's unreliability as skilled workers and, especially, their inability to hold positions of authority.

Construing menopause as a deficiency disease has led, in the United States, to widespread prescriptions of long-term hormonal replacement therapy for specific symptoms, such as hot flashes, night sweats, and vaginal dryness; for diffuse symptoms, such as depression, sleeplessness, fatigue, and sexual disinterest; and for prevention of heart disease and osteoporosis. For an individual woman, short-term hormonal use might be a useful remedy for extremely discomforting symptoms, but long-term use carries the risk of breast and uterine cancer. For women in general, the connotation of menopause as a lack of the crucial mark of womanhood (potential for procreation) undercuts the status of older women as full human beings.

Cross-cultural and cross-national studies give evidence of contrasting views of menstruating women and women who have completed their childbearing. In some cultures, menstruating women have an aura of spiritual and creative power. Similarly, in countries that mark the passage of life transitions ritually and socially, the onset and cessation of menstruation are important events in that they change a woman's status—from child to marriageable woman, from mother to respected elder.

Feminist critiques of the biomedical model of menstruation and menopause have focused on its negative use in rationalizing the subordinate status of women in Western society. They have also publicized the potential risks and side effects of long-term therapy with antidepressants, tranquilizers, and hormones, as well as the stigmatizing consequences of labeling all women as potentially periodically incapacitated or emotionally out of control. Without denigrating the discomforts and debilities some women experience, they have recommended short-term specific use of medical remedies and the effectiveness of alternative medicine. They have also argued that research on the social psychological and situational aspects of menstruation and menopause would produce fuller knowledge of women's feelings and behavior at "that time of month" and "that time of life."

Notes

1. Not all cycles are ovulatory; anovulatory cycles are common when menses first start and as they are stopping (Foster 1996: 537–40).

2. The exact phrasing of the sociological theorem, from a book by Dorothy Swaine Thomas and W. I. Thomas, is: "If men define situations as real, they are real in their consequences" (1927: 47).

3. Katz Rothman points out that the same adherence to supposedly normal timing of physiological events governs medicalized childbirths (1982: 257–74).

4. Brown Parlee feels that it is not a coincidence that widespread attention began to be paid to PMS as a prevalent woman's illness at the same time that feminism became a significant social movement (1994: 101).

5. For other studies on menstrual synchrony, see Golub (1992: 69–70).

6. Fausto-Sterling used the phrase "hormonal hurricanes" in her chapter on menstruation, the menopause, and female behavior (1985: 90–121).

7. *Feminine Forever* was the name of the book popularizing estrogen use written by Robert Wilson (1966), a gynecologist from New York City who had set up a foundation to promote estrogens that was supported by over a million dollars in grants from the pharmaceutical industry (McCrea 1986: 297). The popular literature at the time estrogen was first widely used in menopause was blunt in its description of the postmenopausal woman. The author of *Everything You Wanted to Know about Sex but Were Afraid to Ask* said in the 1969 edition, "Not really a man but no longer a functional woman, these individuals live in the world of intersex" (quoted in Fausto-Sterling 1985: 111).

8. The standard epidemiological definition of natural menopause is twelve consecutive months of amenorrhea with no other cause; perimenopause was defined as a change in cycle regularity or periods of amenorrhea of eleven months or less (Avis and McKinlay 1995: 46).

9. The comparative statistics on rates of hot flashes and night sweats are:

Japan—15.2%, 3% of 1,104

Manitoba—41.5%, 22.2% of 1,039

Massachusetts—43.9%, 11.3% of 5,505

10. Callahan 1993; Greer 1991; Lock 1993; Martin 1992; Voda et al. 1982.

11. One of the most famous remedies for "female complaints" was Lydia E. Pinkham's Vegetable Compound. First marketed in 1875 out of Mrs. Pinkham's home in Massachusetts, it was manufactured for a hundred years (Stage 1979). Its ingredients were "Unicorn root, Life root, Black cohosh, Pleurisy root, and Fenugreek seed macerated and suspended in approximately 19 percent alcohol" (p. 32). The recommended dosage was three spoonfuls a day.

CHAPTER 6

Genital Surgeries: Gendering Bodies

What is "learned by the body" is not something that one has ... but something that one is. . . . . It is never detached from the body that bears it. (Bourdieu 1990, 73)

In Western culture, women and men willingly undergo cosmetic surgery, such as enlargement of breasts and penises, to physically mold their appearance to fit ideals of feminine and masculine beauty.[1] These practices may lead to infections and systemic damage, but they are undertaken as responses to culturally idealized expectations of how women's and men's bodies should look.[2] Other adults (*transsexuals*) undergo surgical changes of their genitalia in order to change their gender and, in part, their sex.[3]

Such surgical changes, since they are undergone voluntarily by adults, need to be distinguished from genital surgery done on children too young to give informed consent. Genital surgery on children agreed to by adults responsible for them are of three kinds—ritual genital surgeries, routine medical surgeries, and "clarifying" surgeries on infants born with ambiguous genitalia (*intersexuals*). The most common forms of ritual female genital surgery are excision of the clitoris (*clitorectomy)* and the outer lips of the vagina. For males, both ritual and medical genital surgery involve removal of the foreskin of the penis (*circumcision).*[4] Surgery on intersexuals includes medical procedures that reduce or enlarge genital organs to make a more normal-looking clitoris or penis and to open or close the area below to create a vagina or scrotum. The goal of intersexual surgery is to reconstruct

93

genital anatomy to conform to the assigned gender of the child and to acceptable, conventional measurements.

Female ritual genital surgery is a health and human rights issue in many countries of the world, and immigration and asylum seekers have brought these practices to the attention of Western countries. Intersexual surgery and accompanying hormonal treatments are done by plastic surgeons and endocrinologists, and so are fully medical procedures, but they also raise issues of bodily integrity and children's rights. Routine circumcision on newborn male infants that is done by medical professionals raises similar concerns, as the medical procedures are rarely physically necessary. Ritual and routine genital surgery and reconstruction of ambiguous genitalia have the cultural purpose of transforming children and pubescent adolescents into what the community considers proper females and males. These practices create gendered bodies and are part of the continuum of risky and often health-endangering behaviors that are responses to pressures to conform to what the community values for bodily masculinity and femininity (Bourdieu 1990, 66–79).

Female Ritual Genital Surgery

For more than two thousand years, in a broad belt across the middle of Africa, various forms of female genital surgery have been used to ensure women's virginity until marriage and to inhibit wives' desire for sexual relations after marriage, and also for aesthetic reasons. (The excised genitals are considered ugly and masculine-looking.) Childbirth becomes more dangerous because of tearing and bleeding, and there are risks of infection and urinary problems after the procedures and throughout life (Bashir 1997). However, there is no comprehensive data on rates of death or on immediate and long-term physical complications from female genital surgery. A review of the studies that did have data on post-surgery problems found a 4- to 16-percent rate of urinary infections, a 7- to 13-percent rate of excessive bleeding, and a 1-percent rate of septicemia (Obermeyer 1999). Some ritual genital surgeries may increase the transmission of HIV infection, but there have been no systematic studies (Brady 1999).

Hanny Lightfoot-Klein estimated that the number of women living in Africa in the 1980s who had their clitorises and vaginal lips excised was 94 million (1989, 31). In the Sudan, these procedures are done on 90 percent of young girls, and in Mali on 93 percent (Dugger 1996). In Egypt, it is estimated that 75 percent of the families excise their daughters' genitalia

(Ericksen 1995). In 1996, the United States passed a law making all of these procedures illegal, and other Western countries with large immigrant populations from Africa have also done so, despite the clash of cultures (Rahman and Toubia 2000; Winter 1994).

The procedures range from mild *sunna* (removing the tip of the clitoris) to modified *sunna* (partial or total clitorectomy) to infibulation or *pharaonic circumcision*, which involves clitorectomy and excision of outer vaginal lips, scraping the inner layers and suturing the raw edges together to form a bridge of scar tissue over the vaginal opening, leaving a small opening for urination and menstruation.[5] Many women have reinfibulation after childbirth and go through the process over and over again. It is called *adlat el rujal* (circumcision for the man) because it is designed to create greater sexual pleasure for men.[6] Karen Paige Ericksen's interviews with sixty-four mothers and twenty-one operators over a ten-year period in Egypt found that the surgical practices were the same, no matter where they were performed or by whom:

> The sequence of the operation is basically the same in both rural villages and popular quarters of Cairo, whether performed by midwives, barbers, medically trained doctors, or itinerant specialists. . . . When it is performed in a doctor's office, a mild sedative, such as Valium, may be given prior to the operation. Surgical instruments, as well as suturing are used, although no mention was made of postoperative checkups. (1995, 313)

Although one of the main rationales for the surgeries is inhibition of female sexual desires to keep girls virginal and wives chaste, reports of the sexual consequences vary considerably. In Lightfoot-Klein's interviews with women throughout the Sudan who had clitorectomies and infibulation, 90 percent described experiencing full orgasms during intercourse once the period of excruciatingly painful opening through penile penetration was over (1989, 80–102). However, Asma El Dareer's survey of 2,375 women, almost all of whom had had full infibulation, found that only 25 percent experienced sexual pleasure all or some of the time (1982, 48). Anthropologists who have done interviews on African women much more recently argue that sexual pleasure after genital surgery is extremely variable (Leonard 2000a; Obermeyer 1999).

Such interviews reveal considerable commitment by women in African societies to having genital surgeries done on their daughters (Williams and Sobieszyzyk 1997). The women say that natural female genitals are unclean and ugly, and the surgeries create a more pleasing, smooth, and "feminine" genital area (Abusharaf 2001). They also feel that these surgeries are an intrinsic part of gendering female bodies—making them into potential or, if pubescent, adult women. However, not all ritual surgeries have a long tradition. Lori Leonard's firsthand studies in Chad found a village where groups of teenage girls began to go off together to have clitorectomies and a coming-out ceremony, as a voluntary rite of passage, like piercing or tattooing, and without the approval of their parents or the village elders (2000b). Whether they went through with the surgery or not had little effect on their marriageability or friendships. In another village, genital surgery had not been a traditional ritual practice a generation ago, but the procedures and accompanying celebrations were borrowed from nearby tribes by groups of young women. The new coming-of-age fad became entrenched, and after a generation, few girls could forego it without ridicule and ostracism.

When done on children too young to consent, from the viewpoint of the West, female genital surgeries seem like the ultimate in child abuse, but from the perspective of the societies where these practices are deeply part of cultural beliefs, not to cut would be a serious breech of parental responsibility.[7] In the parts of the world where these practices are imbued with religious, moral, and esthetic values, ritual genital surgeries make girls into marriageable women. Ellen Gruenbaum's (2000) five years of fieldwork in the Sudan shows that change is coming from within, through the influence of Islamic activists, the work of community health educators, and the efforts of educated African women. Western outrage and external efforts to stop female ritual genital surgeries often provoke a strong backlash in the countries where these practices are common. This clash of cultural perspectives has led one anthropologist to question whether Western women could ever understand why African women would willingly undergo genital surgery and have it done on their young daughters, any more than African women who have had the surgeries can understand how Western women can live with their ugly genitals (Obermeyer 1999). Although Westerners may be reluctant to criticize women's beliefs and practices in cultures not their own, feminist and human rights policies do condemn patriarchal social structures that control and oppress women, as well as practices such as ritual female genital surgeries when they are part of women's subordination.

Male Ritual and Medical Genital Surgery

Male ritual genital surgery is much older and more widespread than female practices (Gollaher 2000).[8] Where girls undergo ritual genital surgery, boys do, too, in the same age range of infancy to young adulthood. However, there are many societies that do not practice female ritual genital surgery but do remove the foreskins of boy babies and young men. Circumcision is part of male coming-of-age ceremonies in some parts of Africa and is a Jewish and Islamic religious covenant, so many more males than females have undergone ritual genital surgery. Culturally, male and female genital surgeries have very different consequences. They both mark children's gender and sexual status, but for boys these are dominant social positions, while for girls they are subordinate statuses.

In Western societies, circumcision is also done on newborns in hospitals for nonreligious reasons. The United States has the highest rate—about 64 percent; in Canada, about 48 percent of males are circumcised (AAP 1999). Circumcision is uncommon in Asia, South and Central America, and most of Europe. In the United States, rates vary by mother's education level and by racial category, with Whites at 81 percent, Blacks at 65 percent, and Hispanics at 54 percent (Laumann et al. 1997). For older men, those whose mothers had a high school diploma were 2.5 times more likely to be circumcised than those whose mothers had not finished high school; for younger men, the significant factor was whether their mother had a college degree.

The recent debates over male genital surgery from a health point of view present a trade-off of risks and benefits. There are high risks, but also potentially high benefits from circumcision before puberty in sub-Saharan Africa, and low risks but few benefits from circumcisions on male infants in Western hospitals.

For the past decade, there have been reports in epidemiological and medical journals about the possible link between circumcision and HIV transmission. When the AIDS epidemic burgeoned in Africa, researchers noted that there was a lower incidence in areas where male ritual genital surgeries were common than where men were not circumcised (Caldwell and Caldwell 1996; Halperin and Bailey 1999). Two comprehensive reviews of twenty-eight studies published up to 1999 on the effect of male circumcision where heterosexual transmission is the predominant mode of infection found a significantly reduced risk of HIV infection in circumcised men—by at least half, and more in particularly high-risk populations (O'Farrell and Egger 2000; Weiss et al. 2000). These studies were done on populations of men in sub-Saharan Africa. An earlier report from Nairobi, Kenya, found a one-third reduction of risk of HIV transmission among women whose husbands or long-term male partners were circumcised (Hunter et al. 1994). Far fewer studies have been done on HIV transmission rates and circumcision in men who have sex with men, but the data have indicated similar reductions in risk (Kreiss and Hopkins 1993).

There seem to be several reasons for this protection (Szabo and Short 2000). One is that genital sores and sexually transmitted diseases are more prevalent in men with foreskins, and these enhance the transmission of the AIDS virus. Second, the foreskin contains a high density of cells that have been identified as the possible primary target for HIV transmission. Third, the foreskin itself is vulnerable to the minilesions and ulcerations that are the sites of entry of the virus. Social variables that might be playing a part in the connection between circumcision and lower risk of HIV infection, such as Muslim religion, did not affect the results (Weiss et al. 2000).

Since the lowered risk rates occur primarily with men who had ritual circumcisions before puberty, no one is suggesting that all men in high-risk populations should immediately be circumcised, but there are ongoing trial programs for encouraging the spread of the practice to communities where it is not a cultural tradition (Bailey et al. 2000). A report from Tanzania indicates that male circumcision may already be taken up by urban secondary school boys from traditionally noncircumcising ethnic groups (Nnko et al. 2001). Unless there is funding for trained circumcisers, antiseptics, and medication for any consequent complications, the results could be disastrous (Ahmed et al. 1999). In South Africa, there have been reports of botched ritual surgeries on adolescent boys done by unskilled or elderly traditional surgeons, as well as HIV infections from unsterilized scalpels (Cauvin 2001).

The debate over the benefits of removal of the penile foreskin in protecting against HIV transmission in sub-Saharan Africa has gotten mixed into the debate over the benefits and risks of circumcision in preventing urinary tract infections, penile cancer, and sexually transmitted diseases in Western societies. Most of the controversy over circumcision in Western societies is over routine hospital surgeries on newborn males.[9] A risk-benefit analysis of 354,297 such circumcisions over a nine-year period in Washington State found 287 complications immediately following the procedure, or one out of 476 (Christakis et al. 2000). The most common complications are bleeding and localized infections, but there have been reports of accidental amputations—and reattachments (Siegel-Itzkovich 2000).

The Task Force on Circumcision of the American Academy of Pediatrics recently reviewed the medical literature of the past forty years to assess the risks and benefits of such circumcisions (AAP 1999). Their review of the benefits indicated that the rate of urinary tract infections in the first year of life is 7 to 14 of 1000 uncircumcised male infants and 1 to 2 of 1000 circumcised male infants; however, the absolute risk of an uncircumcised male infant developing a urinary tract infection in the first year of life is less than 1 percent. Neonatal circumcision offers some protection from cancer of the penis in later life; here, the overall risk is even lower—9 to 10 cases per year per 1 million men. The report argues that the incidence of urinary tract infection and penile cancer in the United States is too low to warrant routine circumcision of male infants. The commission granted the possibility of protection against transmission of HIV and syphilis, but contended that preventive behaviors would be more effective. The commission recommended that parents be informed of the potential benefits and risks of circumcision and that it is a strictly elective procedure. The AAP Circumcision Policy Statement, which was supported by the American Medical Association, reads:

> Existing scientific evidence demonstrates potential medical benefits of newborn male circumcision; however, these data are not sufficient to recommend routine neonatal circumcision. In circumstances in which there are potential benefits and risks, yet the procedure is not essential to the child's current well-being, parents should determine what is in the best interest of the child. To make an informed choice, parents of all male infants should be given accurate and unbiased information and be provided the opportunity to discuss this decision. If a decision for circumcision is made, procedural analgesia should be provided. (AAP 1999, 686)[10]

Another issue that has been raised by activists against circumcision is that it may diminish sexual sensation. In the nineteenth century, circumcision and clitorectomy were both recommended as deterrents to masturbation, which has led activists to argue that removal of the foreskin must deaden sexual feeling (Zoske 1998). However, data from 1,410 American men aged 18 to 59 who participated in the 1992 National Health and Social Life Survey found that self-identified circumcised men had a slightly lesser risk of experiencing sexual dysfunction, such as inability to have orgasms, especially when older (Laumann et al. 1997). The survey also found that circumcised men engaged in more varied sexual practices and masturbated more, but the variation across ethnic groups suggested that differences were due to social factors, which correlate with likelihood of being circumcised. It is unlikely that there will ever be objective data on the differences in sexual pleasure given and received by men with and without foreskins, since these evaluations are so subjective. As Karen Ericksen Paige predicted a generation ago:

> Men have debated the sexual sensitivity question for centuries. Circumcised men think that they have the more sensitive penises; uncircumcised men think that the constant exposure of the naked glans to clothes and the elements toughens it. Some men think that having a foreskin delays orgasm, giving a man more control; others think just the opposite. This discussion is never going to be settled. Sexual sensitivity appears to be in the mind of a man, not in his foreskin. (1978, 46)

As attention to female ritual genital surgery has grown in Western societies, there has been a parallel movement against male genital surgery as a routine post-birth procedure.[11] Western activists claim female and male "circumcision" are equivalent, since in their view sexual sensation is lost with removal of the penile foreskin, and there are equal risks of infection and subsequent mutilation. They have not, however, organized protests against ritual circumcision on African adolescents and young men. The debate over male genital surgery in the West has not centered on cultural conflicts, but on risk-benefit health issues and costs and on sexual sensitivity.

Ritual circumcision on newborn boys among Jews and on adolescent boys among Muslims has rarely been questioned. Some Jews have called for continuing the ceremony of *b'rit milah* without cutting (Goldman 1998; Kimmel 2001), and a few Jewish and Islamic scholars have also questioned whether the Hebrew Bible and the Qur'an do command that all boys and men be circumcised to be full members of their religious communities (Aldeeb Abu-Sahlieh 1994; Hoffman 1995).[12] The broader questions of bodily integrity and the rights of children to intact genitals are raised by secular anticircumcision activists who want international support.

As with female ritual genital surgery, ritual removal of male foreskins is for the community, not the person. Male circumcision ceremonies indicate a father's loyalty to his lineage elders—"visible public evidence that the head of a family unit of their lineage is willing to trust others with his and his family's most valuable political asset, his son's penis" (Paige and Paige 1981, 147). Both reflect patriarchal ideologies—girls are kept virginal, wives are kept chaste, and boys receive the mark of manhood. As Michael Kimmel says:

Circumcision . . . is the single moment of the reproduction of patriarchy. It's when patriarchy happens, the single crystalline moment when the rule of the fathers is reproduced, the moment when male privilege and entitlement is passed from one generation to the next, when the power of the fathers is enacted upon the sons, a power which the sons will someday then enact on the bodies of their own sons. (2001, 48)

Looking at secular circumcisions from a gender perspective, Joe Zoske (1998) depicts them as psychological rituals that imbue boys at birth with the masculine virtues they will supposedly need as adults—the experience of violence, suppression of pain, and emotional distancing. Since these psychological reactions are even more likely to occur in girls undergoing ritual genital surgery, one wonders at the gendering of such "virtues."

Genital Surgery on Intersexuals

Genital surgery is also done on infants who are born with genitalia that do not look clearly male or female, according to conventional views.[13] About 1.7 percent of all infants are born with anomalies of sex chromosomes, internal reproductive organs, and external genitalia in a variety of combinations, not all of which are visible (Fausto-Sterling 2000, 50–54).[14] In Western societies, infants with ambiguous genitalia are assigned a gender and usually undergo "clarifying" surgery to make their genitals conform to this assignment; they are then brought up in the assigned sex, which may not match their internal organs or sex chromosomes (Dreger 1998; Kessler 1998).

The surgical procedures for dealing with intersex infants were developed in the 1920s and 1930s by a urologist, Hugh Hampton Young (Chase 1998). In the 1950s, John Money, the noted Johns Hopkins sex researcher, and Lawson Wilkins, the founder of pediatric endocrinology, instituted the practices of immediate post-birth intervention, and their protocol was widely adopted in hospitals in the United States. The theory behind the early intervention is John Money's contention that gender identity is not established until the child is two years old. As Cheryl Chase, founder of the Intersex Society of North America, describes the still-used Johns Hopkins model,

[t]he birth of an intersex infant today is deemed a "psychosocial emergency" that propels a multidisciplinary team of intersex specialists into action. Significantly, they are surgeons and endocrinologists rather than psychologists, bioethicists, representatives from intersex peer

support organizations, or parents of intersex children. The team examines the infant and chooses either male or female as a "sex of assignment," then informs the parents that this is the child's "true sex." Medical technology . . . is then used to make the child's body conform as closely as possible to that sex. (1998, 191)

Internal organs and hormonal input are usually left to be treated at adolescence, when the intersexual often must undergo additional extensive surgery along with the medical treatments in order to produce a physiology and anatomy that will match the previously assigned sex and gender (Minto and Creighton 2001).

Gender assignment for intersexuals is a biomedical judgment call. Psychologist Suzanne Kessler interviewed pediatric plastic surgeons working with intersexed infants and found that what sex the child with ambiguous genitalia is assigned depends on the size of the penis/clitoris. According to her research, only if the surgeon feels that he (and it is usually a he) can make an adequate-sized penis will the child be made into a boy; otherwise, the sex assignment will be "female" (Kessler 1998). Kessler points out that this social determination of the sex of the child and its construction through surgery is masked by medical rhetoric. The doctors' message to the parents is that the child has a true sex that is female or male, and that the surgery is needed to make the anomalous genitals match the true sex. In actuality, the sex is a social fiction, because the child usually ends up with a combination of male and female biology but is designated a boy or a girl and socialized in the norms of the assigned gender.

Kessler notes that female and male genitalia vary considerably in size. Commenting on how sex and gender categorization are imposed on very visible variability, Kessler says:

Dichotomized, idealized, and created by surgeons, *genitals mean gender.* A belief in two genders encourages talk about "female genitals" and "male genitals" as homogenous types, regardless of how much variability there is within a category. Similarly, the idea of "intersexed" masks the fact that "intersexed genitals" vary from each other as much as they vary from the more idealized forms. (1998, 132)

In the last few years, there has been an intersex movement that protests against "clarifying" surgery on infants (Chase 1998; Turner 1999).[15] The movement argues that this surgery is genital mutilation that ruins future sexual pleasure. The sexual potentialities of true hermaphrodites with male and female genitalia who are not surgically altered can be gleaned from one of Young's cases.[16] Emma was born in 1937 with a penis-like clitoris as well as a vagina. Raised as a girl, Emma used her penis in sexual relationships with women, and her vagina in sexual relations with her husband. She refused to have vaginal closure and live as a man because it would have meant a divorce and having to get a job. Emma's gender identity was that of a woman; she was physiologically bisexed, and thus able to be heterosexual in her sexual relations with her husband as well as with her women lovers. Emma is another instance of the possibilities of multiple sexualities and genders that are conventionalized by "clarifying" surgery and assignment to one gender.

Activists against genital surgery in infancy or childhood recommend that any surgery be left until adolescence, when informed consent is feasible (Chase 2000; Kipnis and Diamond 1998). Yet even if intersexuals' genitalia are not reconstructed to look female or male at infancy, most will of necessity be gendered (Zucker 1999). A gender-neutral or androgynous or "unisex" person is an anathema in a world where people want to know quickly where to place others they encounter for the first time. Social identities are gendered identities; identity papers and bureaucratic records document gender over and over again. Western societies have only two genders, "man" and "woman." Genitalia can be female, male, or ambiguous. Others will assume that the body beneath feminine or masculine clothing has appropriate genitalia—"cultural genitals" (Kessler and McKenna 1985). But since our worlds are so divided by gender, and genitalia are the physical signals of gender, it is not surprising that parents of intersex infants feel they have no choice but to let surgeons construct appropriate-looking genitalia. In their eyes, it would be psychologically damaging for a child to grow up with ambiguous or wrong-looking genitals, which could lead to shaming by peers and rejection by potential sexual partners.

A progressive but perhaps utopian alternative, notes Kessler, would be to view genital variations "as an expansion of what is meant by female and male" (Kessler and McKenna 1985, 131). She is speaking of physical variety, but, as we have seen in this chapter, there is much cultural variety as well—males with and without foreskins, females with and without clitorises and vaginal lips and with open and covered vaginas.

The underlying purpose of genital surgery is to create conformity and uniformity. Genitals are supposed to look "normal" and give a clear signal about the person's sex/gender. Genitals are cultural, because they do not necessarily conform to hormonal or genetic sex. To look different in the locker room (the site always given as the source of danger) is to be stigmatized (Preves 1998). Here again, medicine serves society. The intersex child undergoing "clarifying" genital surgery is actually undergoing operations of social control that perpetuate the conditions of gender conformity.

Politics of Genital Surgery

Female ritual surgeries that remove the clitoris, the main source of sexual sensation in women, are much like the surgeries done on intersex children with large clitorises/small penises. Since it is easier to cut off "excess" than to build up a "lack," many intersex children are feminized, with "good-looking" but desensitized genitalia. Despite the obvious similarities between female ritual genital surgery and intersex surgery, Western feminist protesters against "female genital mutilation" have not joined in the protests against clitorectomies on intersexual babies. In the United States, the Federal Prohibition of Female Genital Mutilation Act specifically excluded "medicalized clitorectomies" on intersex children. Cheryl Chase says the contrasting horrific images of ritual surgery in Africa in the lay press and the objectified clinical images of intersex surgery in medical texts mask an ideological message: "These representations all manifest a profound othering of African clitorectomy that contributes to the silence surrounding similar medicalized practices in the industrialized West. 'Their' genital cutting is barbaric ritual; 'ours' is scientific. Theirs disfigures; ours normalizes the deviant" (1998, 206). Intersex "deviants" need to be "corrected," she goes on, because they "call into question the assumed relation between genders and bodies and demonstrate how some bodies do not fit easily into male/female dichotomies" (p. 208).

The opposite focus occurs in the movement against male genital surgery; it is an effort to stop circumcision of male infants in developed countries. The main target is routine medical circumcisions. The movement activists claim that routine circumcision on newborn infants has only potential benefits in preventing infections, including HIV, and cancers in the man and his women partners, but there are immediate risks of botched surgeries and infections. As for religious reasons, there are few advocates of Jewish (b'rit shalom) rituals without cutting (Goldman 1998) or claims that circumcision is not intrinsic to Islam (Aldeeb Abu-Sahlieh 1994). Western movements against medical circumcision in male infants have not become involved with African ritual circumcision of young men, although these have a documented higher risk of infections, mutilations, and death than those done in Western hospitals (Ahmed et al. 1999; Cauvin 2001).

Genital surgery may have similar outcomes, but the reasons for the surgery justify separate politics. Ritual surgery is done on young girls, often without their consent, to control their sexuality and make them properly "feminine." Subordinate social status and lack of civil rights are as much a political issue as the genital surgery. Ritual surgery on male infants or adolescent boys as part of religious ceremonies is also done without their consent, but makes the boy part of a superior group within Judaism and Islam. In Africa, ritual surgery on male adolescents is part of an eagerly undergone initiation which includes weeks away from home to learn men's roles and behavior as well as to have the culminating removal of the foreskin, marking the boy a man. In the United States, circumcision of newborn boys in hospitals is a medical procedure, with debates over its health benefits and risks and its effects on sexual sensation. Genital surgery on intersex children has elements of female ritual surgery in its imposition on children and goal of bodily gendering, but like routine removal of foreskins in Western hospitals, it is a debatable medical procedure.

What unites these types of genital surgeries is that they are all culturally constructed gendering practices. The most recent joint efforts against them are in the name of human rights and the rights of children, for "genital integrity."[17] To be successful, the coalition movements against genital surgery will need to address cultural conflicts and the gender questions embedded in those conflicts—questions of gender identity, how gendered bodies should look, and genitals as gender markers.

Summary

Genital surgeries are done on newborns and young children without their consent and on adolescents under peer and parental pressure as part of coming-of-age rituals. Girls undergo clitorectomies and removal of the outer lips of the vagina to be marriageable and feminine, according to their culture's views of chastity and how women's bodies should look. In the same cultural groups, boys undergo removal of the penile foreskin (circumcision) to become a man. Circumcision of males eight days after birth or before puberty is part of Jewish and Islamic religious covenants. In Western societies, particularly the United States and Canada, circumcision of newborn boys has been a routine medical procedure. Genital surgeries are also done on children born with ambiguous genitalia (intersexuals) to make them look more like clitorises or penises, depending on the chosen gender.

In the last twenty-five years, all of these procedures have come under fire from health care professionals and activists in organized human rights movements. Those against these genital surgeries have argued that they are unnecessary traumatizing mutilations that reduce sexual sensation and cause serious immediate and long-term complications. Countering these views, supporters cite the importance of long-standing cultural and religious traditions and identification as a man or woman. Those in favor of circumcision cite the medical benefits—potential protection against urinary tract infections, penile cancer and cervical cancer in female partners, and lowered risk of HIV infection. The arguments for "clarification" of the genitals of intersex infants argue that no child can remain genderless in gendered societies, and that the genitals, as the visible sign of gender, should look clearly female or male.

Most recently, the movements against genital surgeries of all kinds have joined forces under the banner of genital integrity, human rights, and rights of children. The debates, like the procedures, are deeply imbued with the meanings of what it is to have the body of a proper girl, boy, woman, or man. The problem is that these meanings differ by culture, religion, and deeply held ideas about the aesthetics and physiology of genitalia and sexuality. The procedures are therefore likely to be done even in the face of the criticism and legal restrictions that result from activist opposition.

NOTES

1. See Bordo 1993, 1999; Davis 1995; Kaw 1998; Luciano 2001.

2. The visual idealization of bodies newly available to laypeople and professionals on the net and in CD-ROM format is usually a White, Westernized body (Moore and Clarke 2001).

3. Transsexuals change the anatomical and bodily part of their sex (many female-to-male transsexuals have hysterectomies and mastectomies as well as genital surgery), but their chromosomes remain XX or XY. The hormones used to counteract the masculinizing or feminizing effects of the internal systems alter their secondary sex characteristics—skin texture, musculature, distribution of body fat, hair growth, breasts. The management of "gender dysphoria" by surgery and hormones is another example of the problematic results of medicalization (Nelson 1998).

4. Another practice, subincision, where the penis is cut through and flattened and urination is subsequently done squatting, occurs only among Australian Aborigines (Montagu 1974).

5. See descriptions in Lightfoot-Klein 1989: 32–36.

6. A comparable procedure in Western obstetrical practice is episiotomy (an incision in the area between the vagina and anus routinely done during childbirth to prevent tearing) and tight suturing after the birth to restore the vagina to its prebirth dimensions (Rothman 1982: 58–59).

7. For discussions of the cultural conflicts, see Abusharaf 2001; Gruenbaum 2000; Shell-Duncan and Hernlund 2000; James 1994, 1998; Leonard 2000a; Obermeyer 1999; Shwerder 2000; van der Kwaak 1992.

8. Penile surgery on two young men is depicted on an Egyptian tomb from 4000 B.C.E. (Paige 1978).

9. In the United States, estimates are that 1.2 million newborn males are circumcised annually at a cost of between $150 to $270 million. Most insurance plans and Medicaid cover the procedure when done in hospitals (AAP 1999).

10. For a protest, see Schoen et al. 2000.

11. Some of the organizations involved are the National Organization of Circumcision Information Resource Centers (NOCIRC), National Organization to Halt the Abuse and Routine Mutilation of Males (NOHARMM), Stop Infant Circumcision Society (SICSOCIETY), Doctors Opposing Circumcision (DOC), Brothers United for Future Foreskins (BUFF), National Organization of Restoring Men (NORM), and RECover a Penis (RECAP). There is an informational Web site, CIRC (Circumcision Reference Library), and on on-line journal, *Circumcision,* edited by Robert Van Howe, M.D. As a counter, circumcisioninfo.com presents "circumcision information explained by doctors, medical establishments, and researchers."

12. For a critical review of the anticircumcision movement from a Jewish perspective, see Levenson 2000.

13. A review of depictions of genitalia in anatomy texts reveals the erasure of variety and, until the feminist movement, no depiction of the anatomy of the clitoris (Moore and Clarke 1995).

14. Some genetic anomalies can be identified prenatally, but their effects may not be accurately predictable, making the decision about whether to continue the pregnancy very difficult (Abramsky et al. 2001).

15. Although there has been some shared activism with genetic sex-variation groups, intersexuals have developed their own more confrontational organization, the Intersex Society of North America, which has a Web site and publishes an on-line newsletter, *Hermaphrodites with Attitude* (Chase 1998). Its goal is to stop genital surgery on infants and to make intersex people more visible to the public.

16. The story of Emma is described in Chase 1998, pp. 190–91, and in Fausto-Sterling 2000, pp. 42–43.

17. The National Organization of Circumcision Information Resource Centers (NOCIRC) and NOCIRC of Australia sponsored the Sixth International Symposium on Genital Integrity, "Safeguarding Fundamental Human Rights in the 21st Century," in Sydney in December 2000. The program covered Jewish and medical male genital surgeries and ritual female surgery. It did not include surgery on intersexuals or Islamic ritual circumcision. NOCIRC and SICSOCIETY (Stop Infant Circumcision) sponsored a Gender Integrity Awareness Week in

Washington, D.C., in April 2001 to bring attention to their cause and to lobby for inclusion of equal protection for males in the law outlawing female genital mutilation. The public information tables included intersex activists, but they were not on the program for the simultaneous Seventh Annual Symposium on Genital Integrity: A New Awareness.

CHAPTER 7

A Modern Plague: Gender and AIDS

And the gay disease, which came to be known as . . . AIDS, slowly ate its way through those new populations, women and their children, hidden and quiet and savage. (Nechas and Foley 1994, 88)

The spread of the epidemic of AIDS (Acquired Immunodeficiency Disease), like the plagues of the past, reflects cultural practices, economics, and politics. When AIDS first surfaced in the United States in 1981, it was identified in the media and medical literature as an epidemic of urban, gay, mostly White middle- and upper-class men.[1] Thought to be caused by promiscuity and high living, it was called GRID (gay-related immune disease). AIDS then became visible in heterosexual women, with clear indications that it was spread through any form of sexual intercourse and that marriage and long-term relationships were no protection. When hemophiliacs who use blood replacement therapy routinely began to get AIDS, the search narrowed to a source that could be transmitted by blood as well as semen.[2] Needle-using drug abusers then proved to be particularly vulnerable, since they contracted AIDS through sharing needles and through sexual exchanges for drugs by both men and women, as well as from partners in long-term relationships. When the AIDS epidemic spread throughout Africa, India, and Asia, it was primarily through heterosexual transmission, along "truck routes"—the paths of transient men seeking work or working as drivers, stopping to have sex with prostitutes, and returning home to infect their wives, who then gave birth to AIDS-infected children.

109

Today, throughout the world, AIDS is known to be a viral infection that produces weakened immune responses and thus extreme vulnerability to other (*opportunistic*) infections. It has become a worldwide epidemic (*pandemic*) of poor men, women, and children, most of whom are Black, Hispanic, or Asian. In all countries, confronting AIDS has repeatedly demonstrated the challenges of diagnosing, treating, and stemming an epidemic in the face of homophobia, racism, sexism, and deeply entrenched economic divisions. Global experiences of AIDS also offer promising illustrations of how marginalized groups (gays and lesbians, women, and people of color) can band together and through the power of social movements transform public health policies and practices.

Biomedically, AIDS is caused by a virus, HIV-1, which enters the cells of the immune system and destroys their capability to fight diseases (Abimiku and Gallo 1995). Although people may live for years with the HIV virus in their bodies, those whose immune systems are severely weakened get infections that cause pneumonia, blindness, diarrhea, and brain deterioration (the symptoms of full-blown AIDS), from which they die. Combinations of drugs can delay the development of AIDS symptoms and produce remissions, so that for those with access to the treatment, it is now a chronic disease instead of a death sentence. The regimen, however, is complicated and expensive, and the drugs can produce major side effects. Most recently, a combination of therapies given immediately after risky sexual or injection exposure to HIV has proved promising in preventing infection (Kahn et al. 2001).

Physiological vulnerability to becoming infected varies, so that not everyone who is exposed becomes HIV-positive or rapidly develops AIDS symptoms. The discovery in 1996 of a genetic mutation that prevents the virus from locking onto cells means that a considerable number of people throughout the world have a built-in protection against HIV infection and an even larger number a delay in breakdown of their immune systems (Dean et al. 1996; Liu et al. 1996).[3]

Socially, AIDS has been a hydra-headed epidemic, surfacing at different times in different populations, with different paths of transmission. As with other aspects of health and illness, a gender analysis focusing on sexual stereotypes and structural inequities between men and women is indispensable to understanding the AIDS picture. In every country, women with AIDS tend to be more socially and economically disadvantaged than men— younger, poorer, less educated, and less employed than men with AIDS. In consequence, women do not have the same access to HIV testing, counseling, and new treatments. In the United States, the decline of new AIDS cases over the past ten years was two times greater for men than for women.[4]

In this chapter, we explore the global social context of HIV transmission and the health care of those with AIDS. Using a gender analysis, we look at the demographics of the disease, outline the risks of getting and transmitting the virus, the care and social support for those who have the symptoms of AIDS, and the implications of the social and cultural construction of the infection and the disease.[5] Keeping in mind the heterogeneous environments and populations that confront AIDS, we investigate both the local and global gender effects of the epidemic.

AIDS by the Numbers

UNAIDS collects and compiles statistical estimates of the *incidence* (new cases) and *prevalence* (current cases) of HIV infection and AIDS throughout the world. These statistics are counts of those who are reported to be HIV-positive or who are treated for diseases to which their compromised immune systems make them vulnerable.[6] In the last twenty years, more than 60 million people worldwide have been infected with HIV, with 40 million living with HIV at the end of 2001. Most of them are 15 to 24 years old. Globally, it is the fourth highest cause of death. In sub-Saharan Africa, it is the leading cause of death. With over 3 million new HIV infections in 2001, over 28 million Africans now live with the virus. In Eastern Europe, especially the Russian Federation, the number of new HIV cases has risen very rapidly, with 250,000 new infections in 2001. A million people now live with HIV in that region, with many more expected. In high-income areas, such as North America and parts of Europe and Australia, there has been a resurgence of new cases.[7]

Within the United States, the estimate of people with HIV/AIDS as of 2000 is 920,000, 25 percent of whom are women. AIDS is no more equally distributed among populations in the United States than it is in the rest of the world. African-American women represent only 13 percent of the U.S. female population, but they accounted for 63 percent of new AIDS cases among women in 1999. Women and men with HIV in the United States cluster in different exposure categories. As of 2000, of 35,775 women with HIV, 41 percent had been exposed through heterosexual contact and 20 percent through injection drug use. Of 92,503 men with HIV, 45 percent were exposed by having sex with men and 14 percent through drug use[8] (see table 7.1).

Table 7.1

AIDS and HIV in the United States, by Exposure Category and Sex, 2000

| Exposure category | Cumulative Total | | | | | |
| | HIV[a] | | | AIDS | | |
	Male	Female	Total	Male	Female	Total
Men who have sex with men	41818		41818	348657		348657
Injecting drug user	12686	7033	19719	137650	51592	189242
Men who have sex with men and inject drugs	5752		5752	47820		47820
Haemophilia (Hemophilia)/ coagulation disorder	439	23	462	4847	274	5121
Heterosexual contact	6553	14589	21142	27952	50257	78209
Receipt of blood transfusion, blood components, or tissue	376	415	791	4920	3746	8666
Other/risk not identified	24879	13715	38594	48343	19042	67385
Total	**92503**	**35775**	**128278**	**620189**	**124911**	**745100**

Source: HIV/AIDS Surveillance Report: "U.S. HIV and AIDS Cases Reported Through June 2000." U.S. Department of Health and Human Services, National Center for HIV, STD and TB Prevention.

[a]These HIV figures include only those states with confidential HIV reporting.

Age distribution is also skewed, with over 80 percent of cases of HIV diagnosed between the ages of 20 and 44 (see table 7.2). Demographic reports of illness and death rates in Africa, India, and Asia similarly indicate that AIDS decimates young adults, in some villages wiping out an entire generation, leaving orphan children and elderly grandparents. In South Africa, the AIDS epidemic has hit young women particularly hard, so that more women are dying at age 25 than at age 60 (Dorrington et al. 2001).

Although there were reports of HIV infection in women as early as 1982 in the United States, it took years before the medical profession acknowledged that women got AIDS.[9] At the beginning of the epidemic, the focus of attention in clinical trials and the mass media was on women's potential to infect men and babies, not on their potential to be infected. Researchers subsequently found that in heterosexual relationships, women are more vulnerable than men are—the male-to-female rate of

Table 7.2

U.S. HIV Cases by Age at Diagnosis, through June 2000[a]

Age at diagnosis	Male	Female	Total	%
Under 5	772	835	1607	1
5-12	252	204	456	0
13-19	2292	2970	5262	4
20-24	11471	6053	17524	13
25-29	18778	7149	25927	20
30-34	20786	7098	27884	21
35-39	17021	5474	22495	17
40-44	10866	3437	14303	11
45-49	5729	1803	7532	6
50-54	2848	813	3661	3
55-59	1352	458	1810	1
60-64	714	235	949	1
65 or older	646	285	931	1
Total	93527	36814	130341	100%

Source: HIV/AIDS Surveillance Report: "U.S. HIV and AIDS Cases Reported Through June 2000." U.S. Department of Health and Human Services, National Center for HIV, STD and TB Prevention.

[a] These HIV figures include only those states with confidential HIV reporting.

transmission is much higher than the female-to-male rate (Padian et al. 1987; Padian et al. 1991). In 2000, global estimates were that roughly 55 percent of adults living with HIV/AIDS are women.[10] As a result, understanding and preventing mother-to-child transmission is a priority in the international AIDS prevention community.

Widely accepted sexual categories may not be useful for estimating the prevalence of HIV infection. Sexual identity does not accurately predict sexual behavior since many self-identified heterosexual men and women, lesbians, and gay men engage in "cross-over" relationships (Goldstein 1995; Scheper-Hughes 1994).

Familiar groupings, such as "prostitutes," cover a heterogeneous range of women, men, and children who sell a variety of sexual services (Patton 1994, 48–59). The term blurs important risk variables, such as identity as a professional sex worker, a group more likely to encourage condom use than those bartering sex for drugs (Moore 1997).[11] Children who sell sex are the most vulnerable of all, since they are unlikely to make any demands on their customers, and they often suffer vaginal and anal tears that make HIV infection probable. Particularly at risk have been poor young women and street children recruited to the sex industry in Latin America and Southeast Asia (Bond 1992; Wawer et al. 1996). Categories of those most at risk, such as needle-sharing drug users and their sexual partners, are usually summations of individual cases; they do not provide data on the community institutions and social networks that can encourage or discourage risk behaviors (Crystal and Jackson 1992; Kane and Mason 1992; Neigus et al. 1994).

In the United States and Europe, the availability of drugs to reduce or delay the appearance of opportunistic diseases in those infected with HIV has led to longer life spans, but also to the relaxation of vigilance against risky sexual behavior. As a result, HIV infection rates have risen where they had previously dropped or stabilized.[12] In addition to this rise in new cases, the longer life spans add to the number of people living with AIDS, and the lower mortality rate increases the number of people who can transmit the HIV virus.[13]

There is also a possible "second wave" of infection among young homosexual men who feel that AIDS is now treatable, so they are less vigilant about safer sex practices. A similar denial of vulnerability may be occurring among young women as well. According to data from 25 U.S. states' reports, the rate of HIV infection from heterosexual sex among teenage girls rose by nearly 117 percent between 1994 and 1998, and there was a 90-percent increase due to injection drug use (Lee and Fleming 2001).

These statistics on HIV and AIDS are outcomes of people's behavior in social networks and gendered relationships. Understanding gendered sociocultural meanings of what it is to be a man (e.g., multiple anonymous sexual encounters) and what it is to be a woman (e.g., to produce several children) is imperative in charting the terrain of the AIDS pandemic. Equally important is attention to the social statuses of those most at risk— an interweaving of sexual stigmas, poverty, restricted health care resources, and political powerlessness. To understand what these statistics mean for the people affected and their families, and what health care and public health policies should be built on them, we must look at the social contexts of transmission, risk, and prevention.

Social Paths of Transmission

Everyone is not at the same risk for AIDS. The transmission of HIV infection clusters by racial and ethnic group, social class, gender, sexual behavior, intravenous drug use, and access to medical treatment for other sexually transmitted diseases. In rural southern United States, where Black women are disproportionately infected with HIV, joblessness, substance abuse, teenage pregnancy, sexually transmitted diseases, inadequate schools, minimal access to health care, and entrenched poverty conspire to thwart the progress that has been made among other high-risk groups, particularly gay men (Sack 2001).

Epidemiologists now talk of Pattern I and Pattern II countries, with different types of HIV transmission profiles and core groups—"small numbers of highly sexually active individuals with large numbers of partners who mix with individuals who would otherwise be deemed at a low risk of infection" (Bloor 1995, 16). Pattern I countries are in the developed or Westernized world. The main sources of transmission are unprotected anal intercourse and use of unsterile equipment to inject drugs; most of those with HIV infection or AIDS are men; the core groups are men who have unprotected sex with men, and men and women drug users who share needles and syringes. Pattern II countries are in the developing part of the world, mainly Africa, Asia, and India. The main source of transmission is heterosexual intercourse; almost half of those with HIV infection or AIDS are women; the core groups are women who sell or barter sexual services and migrant men workers, such as truck drivers and workers who leave their wives to run the family farm while they seek employment in the city (Bloor 1995, 10–54). In these parts of the world, "one can trace the evolution of the epidemic with eerie accuracy simply by comparing traffic patterns moving out of major cities with the rates of infection of people who live along the way" (Specter 2001, 77).

As an exposure category, injection drug use is a social behavior with multiple associated stigmas. It is not just needle users who are at risk of HIV through sharing a used syringe; sexual partners of needle users, often unaware of their partner's drug use, are also at risk. Long-term relationships are embedded in tightly interlocked networks whose norms, based on trust and loyalty, may foster high-risk behavior. As an intensive study in an area in New York City with a high incidence of HIV infection found:

> Fully 70% of the drug injectors interviewed . . . injected or shared syringes with a spouse or sex partner, a running partner, or with friends or others

whom they knew. . . . [T]he social relationship of drug injectors with members of their risk network were often based on long-standing multiplex relationships, such as those based on kinship, friendship, marital and sexual ties, and economic activity. The intertwining of drug using relationships with these other social relationships implies that attempts to reduce HIV risk behavior among drug injectors may have ramifications for these other relationships, which in turn may either facilitate or hinder the success of such attempts. (Neigus et al. 1994, 75–76)

Multiple research studies from the United States, Sweden, Australia, and the Netherlands have demonstrated that needle-exchange and drug-treatment programs decrease the rate of HIV infection (Espinoza et al. 1988; Hartgers et al. 1992). Not only are users able to obtain free and clean syringes, but they can also get information about safer sex and drug treatment.[14]

The U.S. criminal justice system, most specifically the administration of prisons and jails, has created an environment rife with HIV risks. Even though we may think of HIV and prison as a men's health issue, since in 1999 almost 95 percent of the prison population was men,[15] many of those who are released from prison with HIV infections carry the disease to their women partners. Men do come to prison already infected with HIV, but if they are not, risk behaviors, such as injecting drugs, unprotected sex, and tattooing, increase the likelihood of exposure while incarcerated. These risk behaviors are illegal for prisoners, but they do occur, consensually and forced. The increased prevalence and incidence of HIV in prisons has been identified in several countries in addition to the United States—Norway, Ireland, France, Germany, Argentina, Brazil, and Honduras.[16]

A U.S.-based longitudinal research project aimed at men in prison and their women partners found that prison policies do not provide access to condoms or clean syringes; yet half of men inmates reported a history of injecting drugs (Zack and Grinstead 2001; also see Polych and Sabo 2000). This study further showed that most inmates, upon release, return to a woman partner and have unprotected sex. Their partners usually know the risks of HIV, but if they were monogamous, they do not consider themselves in danger because they are not aware of the increased HIV risks with incarceration. Peer-based interventions after leaving prison have been effective in increasing use of condoms and reducing injecting drugs (Grinstead et al. 1999).[17]

Safer Sex

"Safe sex" has entered the language of HIV prevention. Actually only *safer* sex, it consists of a collection of technical devices and hands-on know-how transmitted to (and among) professionals, partners, peers, and sex workers (Moore 1997). Safer sex is thus a form of embodied knowledge (Haraway 1989). The estimation of risks of sexual practices is usually read against the shield of abstinence, but it is unrealistic to expect abstinence in a long-term relationship, even if one partner is HIV-positive and the other negative. In any relationship, estimates of risk of sexual practices are inevitably subjective and prone to negotiation with partners.

Safer sex is usually achieved by the use of latex devices. Most sexual practices that involve the exchange of body fluids can be modified and made less risky by using barriers. For example, male and female condoms are used for anal and vaginal intercourse and oral sex, latex gloves can protect hands, and dental dams or saran wrap can make oral sex less risky. (See table 7.3 for a list of risks of sexual practices.)

Male condoms are widely known to be the best protection against HIV infection, as well as against other sexually transmitted diseases. But they are infrequently used in long-term heterosexual or homosexual relationships because "condom use may be perceived as signaling a lack of trust in one's partner and because a partner toward whom one has affectionate feelings is usually not perceived as a potential source of the disease, regardless of the risk history of the individual" (Kelly 1995a, 346). As one young woman said, "We've entered a period where mistrust equals responsibility, where fear signifies health" (Daum 1996, 33).

For men, safer sex is in their own hands, literally, if they put on condoms. But women find it very difficult to get their men sexual partners to use condoms if they don't want to (Wermuth et al. 1992). Women have feared violent reactions to their insistence on condom use, as well as to getting tested (Cooper 1995, 287). So that women could have some control, devices specifically for their use have been produced. The female condom is a loose tube made of polyurethane. One end is closed with an internal moveable ring, and there is an external stable ring incorporated into the tube. The internal ring is placed on the woman's cervix, and the external ring covers the outer area of the vagina, the labia. The penis, not necessarily completely erect, is inserted into the tube during vaginal intercourse. This one-time only device can be inserted prior to intercourse.

The female condom has the potential to save money in treatment of HIV and other sexually transmitted diseases, as well as lives, but the

Table 7.3

Sex Practices, Safety and Risks

Safe or Very Low Risk Practices
Sensual massage
Hugging, cuddling, snuggling
Mutual self-masturbation
Social/dry kissing or tongue kissing on anywhere but mouth, genitals and anus
Dry humping
Showering together
Phone sex, computer sex
Fantasy
Flirting
Sadomasochistic games without bruising or bleeding
Viewing pornography (movies, books, live dancing)

Possibly Safe or Possibly Risky Practices[a]
French kissing
Anal intercourse with latex condom
Vaginal intercourse with latex condom
Fisting with a latex glove
Oral sex with latex barriers/ oral sex on a man without ejaculation
Fingering with latex barrier
Water sports — contact with urine (not in open cut or wound)

Possibly Unsafe Practices[b]
Oral sex without a latex barrier (especially during menstruation)
Fingering without a latex barrier
Fisting without a latex barrier
Sharing sex toys without latex barriers

Unsafe Practices
Anal intercourse without a condom
Vaginal intercourse without a condom
Masturbating with other's body fluid
Rimming without a latex barrier
Blood contact
Oral sex on a woman during her period

Adapted from C. Winks and A. Semans. 1994. *The Good Vibrations Guide to Sex.* Pittsburgh, PA: Cleis Press.

[a,b] It is within the "Possibly Safe" and "Possibly Unsafe" categories that innovations and controversial safer sex ideas are constantly being reformulated. The modifier "possibly" creates a space for judgment to rest with the individual and protects against the potential liability of administering lethal advice.

current prices of two to three dollars apiece has made them inaccessible for many women (Marseille et al. 2001).[18] Researchers in Thailand found that when male and female condoms were both promoted and made accessible to sex workers, there was an increase in the number of protected sexual encounters (Fontanet et al. 1998), but the female condom is not particularly well accepted. Sex workers in a 1996 study in the San Francisco Bay area criticized the device for being noisy, cumbersome, and expensive (Moore 1997). Comments from those interviewed indicate their objections. Felicia said, "It looks like a colostomy bag. And it is too expensive; I would prefer to use a male condom at 25 cents a pop." Hadley said, "I don't associate that thing with sex."

Although studies show a desire for woman-controlled devices to prevent heterosexual transmission of HIV (Elias and Coggins 2001), there is a question of how much negotiation is needed to use the female condom. A recent study in New York City, Baltimore, and Seattle enrolled 604 women at high risk for STDs and HIV in a randomized controlled trial (Van Devanter et al. 2002). These women were placed in small groups and received training in how to insert the female condom through a video, a clinician's demonstration, and a personal opportunity to practice on a pelvic model. Through interviews and self-administered questionnaires, researchers determined that "female-controlled" may be a misnomer because some negotiation with partners is required. Training was beneficial, but so was confidence in asking for the use of any condom.

Ironically, prevention of HIV transmission has been more successful in commercial sexual behavior than in romantic relationships. Sex workers are more knowledgeable about the techniques and devices of safer sex and more likely to use them. A long-term study of 3,066 women streetwalkers in New York City found a substantial decline in HIV infection in response to an intensive program of distribution of condoms and dental dams, bleach kits, food, and sleeping bags, and counseling and referral to agencies for further help (Whitmore et al. 1996). In his discussion of prostitute women, Michael Bloor notes that "it is one of the ironies of the HIV epidemic that the public health has been preserved by the efforts of one of the most vilified and marginalized groups in society" (1995, 75).

The Gender Politics of Risk and Prevention

Since HIV/AIDS is primarily a sexually transmitted disease, the vulnerability of the penetrated is the essence of probable exposure to HIV infection. In Mexico, Brazil, and in the Asian sex tourism industry, gender and sexual categories are overridden by relationships of power and dominance. Men who define themselves as heterosexual engage in anal and vaginal penetration of men and women lovers, male and female sex workers (who are often very young), and their own wives (Alonso and Koreck 1989; Bloor 1995, 19–24; Parker 1992). Nancy Scheper-Hughes, an anthropologist who has done extensive field work in Brazil, blames

> the special place of a liberated sexuality in the Brazilian male social imaginary, as an imagined space where everything is permitted, nothing is forbidden, and where sexual sin does not exist. [Anthropologists] note the "catholicity" of sexual tastes and preferences within the Brazilian sexual ideology: for anal/oral sex across all sexual identities; for inter-racial and inter-generational sex; and above all, a fluid and pervasive bisexuality. (1994, 993)

The range of sexual behaviors and gender differences in social power should be kept in mind in any discussion of HIV risk factors.[19]

Whatever the gender composition, the closer the relationship, the less likely the partners are to practice safer sex. The way to change sexual behavior, therefore, may be to foster community norms that "emphasize safer sex as a way for people to show their concern, love, affection, and care for one another" (Kelly 1995a, 346).[20] Nancy Scheper-Hughes would probably say that the "commandments" those infected with HIV in Cuba must swear to in order to live outside the sanitariums they are confined in would be more effective: "To have unprotected sex with an unknowing, uninfected individual is murder. Consensual sex with an uninfected and informed partner is criminal" (1994, 999).

Since the transmission of HIV/AIDS is embedded in relationships, we examine separately those involving women with men, men with men, and women with women. In all of these types of sexual relationships, many of the partners have sex with women and with men, so none should be considered exclusively heterosexual or homosexual.

Men and Women

One of the chief routes of transmission of HIV for women in the United States has been unprotected heterosexual intercourse with infected partners. The transmission rates are disproportionately higher among Black women and Latinas than among White women, in part because they are more likely to live in poor communities with a high incidence of drug use, violence, rape, commercial sex, and multiple partners (Hammonds 1992; Lewis 1995; Nyamathi and Vasquez 1989). Forced sex, which many women experience throughout their lifetime, has been associated with greater risk for HIV infection and less likelihood of HIV testing (Molitor et al. 2000).

In the early 1990s, women sex workers were accused of spreading the disease (Campbell 1991; King 1990), but then came reports that a woman is much more vulnerable to HIV infection from intercourse with an HIV-positive man than a man is from an HIV-positive woman—an ejaculation is an excellent conveyer of the virus, and semen stays in the vagina for days (Nicolosi et al. 1994; Padian et al. 1987; Padian et al. 1991). A study of 379 monogamous heterosexual White couples in their thirties who were followed over five years found that among the 72 men whose woman partner was HIV-positive, only one got infected, while 20 percent of the 307 women with HIV-positive male partners did (Padian et al. 1991).

It is harder for some women to insist on male condom use or safer sex practices in love relationships than in casual encounters or when male partners are paying for sex. In a study of 377 women of varied race and class who lived in Florida, 74 percent of the 268 with a main partner said they used condoms in less than half of the times they had vaginal or anal intercourse, while 70 percent of the 109 with client partners reported condom use more than half the time (Osmond et al. 1993). This study also found that when condoms were used, it was overwhelmingly because the woman made the decision and her partner agreed to it, and that women were more assertive and men more compliant when sex was for sale. However, the African-American women in the Florida study were much more successful in getting their main partners to use condoms than the White women or Latinas (86 percent of the time compared to an average for the whole group of 26 percent); they were in more unstable relationships and were less dependent economically on their main partners.

A study of 185 African-American and White adolescents aged fourteen to nineteen with a steady heterosexual partner found a similar pattern of lesser commitment to the relationship and more power to negotiate condom use among younger White girls and older African-American girls who felt at risk for AIDS (Gutiérrez et al. 2000). Carole Campbell criticizes the premises of risk-control programs that put the onus on women to learn how to negotiate condom use: "These strategies serve to reinforce the idea that safer sex is a female concern and responsibility. They fail to address the issue of why women should even have to negotiate safer sex in the first place. That is, they fail to address why safer sex is not a male concern and

responsibility" (1995, 205). In recognition of women's relative powerlessness in heterosexual encounters, they are held less accountable than men
are for getting AIDS from unprotected consensual sex (Borchert and
Rickabaugh 1995).

Despite the recognized difficulty women have of getting their male
partners to use condoms, all of the emphasis in Western-oriented prevention programs is based on education and individual responsibility.
Knowledge about HIV transmission and risk can be high among young
people but condom use low because of social norms about sexual behavior (MacPhail and Campbell 2001). In some communities, knowledge and
interpretation of risk are often both correct and incorrect, and the use of
protective devices is equally mixed (London and Robles 2000).

Men and Men

Within industrialized nations, during the mid 1980s, the tireless prevention and awareness work of community-based organizations, including
lesbian/gay/bisexual and transgender groups, encouraged prevention and
helped halt the massive devastation of AIDS among gay men. The incidence
of HIV/AIDS among White gay men fell between 1994 and 1998.[21] Since
the late 1990s, however, sexual risk-taking has been on the rise among
young men who have sex with men (Ekstrand et al. 1999). A recent survey
of gay men in San Francisco found that those who said they always used a
condom during anal sex dropped to 49.7 percent in 2000 from 69.6 percent
in 1994. During the same period, men having unprotected anal sex with
more than one partner increased to 48.8 percent from 23.4 percent (Goode
2001). A study conducted in six U.S. cities from 1998 to 2000 found that the
rate of new HIV infections among the men in the study who were between
23 and 29 years old was 4.4 percent: 2.5 percent among Whites, 3.5 percent
among Hispanics, and 14.7 percent among Blacks. Among men who were
knowledgeable about safer sex practices, 46 percent reported having unprotected anal intercourse. In this study, Black men who have sex with men
were five times more likely to become HIV-infected than their White coun-
terparts.[22]

Although many feminists have deplored the powerlessness of women
in trying to get male lovers and husbands to use condoms, so that "romantic sex . . . is *unsafe* sex" (Osmond et al. 1993, 116), studies of gay men have
found the same phenomenon—"penetrative sex occurs most frequently
with a regular sexual partner and, as in heterosexual relationships, is seen

as emblematic of intimacy, love and trust; sex with regular partners is much more likely to involve unsafe sex than sex with casual partners" (Bloor 1995, 57). Such a division between protected casual sex and unprotected monogamous sex has considerable risk because in both same-gender and cross-gender romantic relationships, individuals overestimate their partner's fidelity as well as ignore their own and their partner's sexual history.

Among gay men in Australia, casual sex with partners picked up in public places is not usually anal-genital; it more likely to be oral sex. Anal-genital sex is more typical of long-term relationships—it conveys trust, intimacy, relatedness, reciprocal give-and-take, and a denial of their own past sexual relationships (Connell and Kippax 1990). The paradox, therefore, is that condoms are least used where they are most needed:

> To the extent that "safe" sex is identified with using condoms for anal sex (a very common understanding), and anal sex is identified with intimacy and relationship, then the less intimate sexuality of the beat [public sexual encounter] may seem not to require precautions. On the other hand, sex in relationships being connected with an ideal of monogamy ("being the only one") may be seen as "safe" *because of the relationship*. Most of the respondents who are currently in couple relationships practice unprotected anal sex with their lovers *whether or not* they are sure their partners have no other sexual contacts. Where the medical definition of prevention conflicts with the social definition of relationships and practices, the social meanings prevail. (Connell et al. 1993, 123; emphasis in original)

Among gay men, casual sex without attachment can be seen as an adoption of dominant masculine norms by a stigmatized group (Kimmel and Levine 1991). Recognizing the glamour of the "stud," one technique of HIV education has been to use "gay heroes"—locally popular gay men—as educators and safe-sex mentors (Kelly et al. 1991). What is taught, however, tends to be filtered through local beliefs, so that men who routinely and intentionally have unprotected anal and oral sex often justify what they do with reasons based on their own interpretations of risky sexual practices (Levine and Siegel 1992). However, peer-based interventions have been successful in reducing the rates of unprotected anal intercourse with both casual partners and boyfriends (Kegeles et al. 1999).

Women and Women

If men who have sex with men have been the group with the highest risk of becoming HIV-positive in the United States, then women who have sex with women should be the group with the lowest risk (Chu and Wortley 1995, 5). The rates of female-to-male transmission are low, so the rates of female-to-female transmission should be even lower. There are two problems with this logic. First, no one really knows the transmission risks of lesbian sexual practices, such as oral-genital contact and the shared use of sex toys (Gómez 1995; Kennedy et al. 1995; Patton 1994, 65–75). Second, it is difficult to conduct research on these specific behaviors because many women who have sex with women do not engage exclusively in one kind of sexual behavior. Women who primarily have sex with women seem to be more at risk when they do have sex with men than women who only have heterosexual relationships—they are less likely to use condoms and more likely to exchange sex for crack cocaine, and also to have other sexually transmitted diseases (Bevier et al. 1995; Gómez 1995).

The risk of HIV infection in woman-to-woman oral sex in particular has been the subject of much debate (O'Hanlan 1995). In many circles, lesbians question the need to use latex dental dams (O'Sullivan and Parmar 1992); they question the actual risks associated with particular practices and attribute the discussion of dangers to AIDS hysteria or a misunderstanding or denigration of lesbian sexual practices. According to one article, "Many lesbians believe it is safe to go down on another woman, except during her menstrual period, and think it is possibly just a societal stigma against their sexual practices that demands use of an artificial barrier" (McMillan 1996, 3). However, Amber Hollibaugh, director of the Lesbian AIDS Project, targets the belief that "true" lesbians don't get AIDS as the source of their possibly greater risk in sexual relationships than female transmission rates would predict (Hollibaugh 1995). She points out that trust and emotional intimacy are the hallmarks of lesbian relationships: "It is hard to imagine, then, how to begin discussing safer sex, negotiating with a lover, HIV and STD protection methods, talking openly about our drug or sex histories" (p. 228). Yet vaginal yeast infections and sexually transmitted diseases *are* passed between women lovers (Bauer and Welles 2001). Without accurate knowledge of what sexual behaviors are dangerous, particularly during menstruation, women who have sex with women *are* at risk: "Lesbianism is not a condom for AIDS" (Hollibaugh 1995, 230).

Mother-to-Child Transmission

One of the most unfortunate outcomes of the AIDS epidemic has been the transmission of the virus to newborns by mothers who carry the infection. Since very often the fathers as well are infected, the children are not only vulnerable to developing AIDS symptoms, but many have been orphaned as well.[23] The risk of mother-to-child transmission is 15 to 25 percent in industrialized countries and 25 to 35 percent in developing countries.[24] This difference is largely attributed to the prevalence of breastfeeding as a significant source of infection.

Since 1994, AZT (an antiretroviral drug) and a lower-cost drug, nevirapine, have been used to cut the risk of transmitting HIV during childbirth. However, most data indicate that breastfeeding must be completely abandoned in order for the drugs to be effective in reducing mother-to-child transmission, since HIV-positive mothers may still expose HIV-negative infants with breast milk. Unfortunately, even when mothers are aware of the dangers of transmission by breastfeeding, there may be no viable alternative food source for infants. In addition, many mothers fear exposure of their HIV-positive status if they do not breastfeed. In Thailand, a simplified AZT regimen given to HIV-infected mothers reduced the rate of HIV transmission from 30 percent to about 10 percent (MMWR 2001). The pilot program included counseling, confidential testing, and free powdered infant formula for a year after the birth.

Within the United States, the related ethical, public health, and private dilemma is whether a woman who knows she is HIV-positive or who is being treated for AIDS symptoms should deliberately become pregnant, or if she does so accidentally, whether she should have an abortion (Pies 1995). The pragmatic answer of many in the U.S. medical community has been an unequivocal "no" to becoming pregnant and "yes" to terminating a pregnancy. But feminist ethicists and advocates for women have pointed out that methods that are more effective than condoms in preventing pregnancy, such as diaphragms, intrauterine devices, and oral contraceptives, not only do not protect against transmission of HIV, they may make transmission more likely by producing vaginal abrasions and changing vaginal secretions (Duerr and Howe 1995; Hutchison and Shannon 1993). Even spermicides can increase the rate of HIV transmission. Sterilization puts an end to fertility. As for obtaining a clinic abortion, it can be financially or physically difficult in general and even more so for HIV-infected women. Drug-induced abortions must be done early, and, as with hormone-based contraception, the drugs may have detrimental effects on HIV-positive women.

On the other hand, there are risks of pregnancy if a woman is HIV-positive or has symptoms of AIDS (Minkoff 1995). There is some evidence that the immune system may be further weakened and the progression of the disease accelerated. Any AIDS treatment must be continued, but unfortunately, the effects of many of the widely used drugs on pregnant women and the fetus are unknown because pregnant (and potentially pregnant) women were, for a long time, excluded from AIDS drug trials (Korvick et al. 1996; McGovern et al. 1994). Even the effects of AZT on pregnant women themselves were not determined in the initial trials.[25]

As with all calculations of risk, many elements go into the procreative decisions of HIV-positive women. The likelihood of transmission of the virus is relatively low and can be lowered further with prenatal administration of AZT.[26] Not all children who are HIV-positive immediately develop symptoms of AIDS, and the armamentarium of treatments is ever-growing. A child has immense intrinsic value, especially in the communities and cultures many HIV-positive women live in, including the wives of hemophiliacs (Jason et al. 1990). The potential father's feelings are an important factor, too (Mbizvo and Bassett 1996).

The most pragmatic question is usually not asked—what is the level of care mothers with AIDS and their children can expect? What level of care for anyone with AIDS?

Living with AIDS

The great breakthrough in the treatment of HIV has been the drug combinations that can substantially slow the progress of HIV growth in those newly infected and reduce HIV levels in those with longer periods of infection. While the virus may still be present in organs and glands, these drugs inhibit viral replication and can stop the virus from weakening the immune system. But even when patients are able to afford the drugs and can integrate the regimen into their lives, it is a challenge for many to consistently comply with complicated schedules. Patient adherence to drug regimens is hampered by drug or alcohol abuse, erratic work schedules, dietary restrictions, and side effects (Chesney 2000). As predicted, resistant strains of the HIV virus have already appeared (Borman et al. 1996). A U.S. and Canadian study conducted during 1999 determined that 14 percent of new HIV cases were infected with drug-resistant strains (Altman 2001).

In industrialized countries, class, color, gender, ethnicity, and drug use—all the stigmata of the lives of people with AIDS—also work against them when they seek medical services. Poor women of color often feel they have fallen through the cracks of the U.S. health care system and social service agencies (Seals et al. 1995). Antonio Coello Novello, a previous Surgeon General of the United States, listed barriers to receiving care: Clinics that are not open during hours they can go, too far from their homes, up flights of stairs they can't climb; no facilities for child care or for buying food for their children or themselves; fragmented care—children in one place, themselves in other, partners someplace else; language barriers; and cultural insensitivity (Novello 1995, xii). It is no wonder, then, that survival rates have been worse for women than men with AIDS in the United States. They come into the medical system later and are poorer, have fewer social supports, may have been heavy drug users, and are often homeless and raped and beaten (Melnick et al. 1994).

While some AIDS patients are struggling to adjust to complicated drug regimens, others are protesting patent laws which have led to the lack of affordable drugs within their national borders. Globally, the primary burden of disease to people living with HIV/AIDS has been the most common infections: tuberculosis, pneumonia, diarrhea, and candida (yeast) infections. These diseases can be treated with anti-infective agents, but these drugs, as well as the antiretroviral drugs for counteracting the virus itself, have been unavailable in generic, cheaper form. Antiretroviral drugs can cost a patient over $10,000 a year and may not be covered by insurance plans (Altman 2000). In African countries, where health care expenditures range from only $1 to at most $200 per capita, it is beyond the means of either public health systems or individuals to finance adequate drug treatments that can strengthen their immune systems and treat the infections and pain of full-blown AIDS.[27]

Recently, some drug companies have succumbed to grassroots as well as international pressure to allow generic makers to market low-cost HIV drugs in Africa and India; some are distributing them free of charge (Pear 2001; Peteren and McNeil 2001). The prospective availability of cheaper or free antiretroviral drugs is not without potentially devastating problems. Uneven distribution and poorly monitored antiretroviral treatment could lead to the rise and transmission of more resistant strains of HIV (Crossette 2001; Specter 2001). Furthermore, in a global market of limited public health funds, the focus on antiretroviral drugs, even at a reduced price, means less funding for education and prevention programs. Distributing condoms that cost pennies is far more effective in the long run than distributing drugs that cost dollars. In India, which has developed a combination of three main AIDS drugs mixed into an inexpensive single tablet that can be taken twice a day, "the simple cost of shipping the drugs around the country and storing them could equal the money the governments spends on treating all other infectious diseases combined" (Specter 2001, 85).

Research for a vaccine that would protect against HIV infection is on-going and may eventually prove to be a turning point in changing a pandemic into an ordinary illness. However, as with so much about AIDS, vaccine research is not without controversy (Collins 2000). First, it is ethically difficult to enroll people in vaccine trials and expose them to HIV when it is unclear if the vaccine will be effective. Second, there is the danger that the focus on vaccine research will limit public and private funds and resources that could go to prevention strategies. Third, the initial distribution and administration of a vaccine is likely to follow the existing social hierarchies with respect to AIDS, so that those at the bottom of the social scale will be targeted as populations to test the vaccine's efficacy and safety, and then those at the top will have the first benefit of its use.

Despite the scientific promise of new drug combinations and the possibility of radical viral load transformations for individuals, caring for millions of people with HIV/AIDS in communities with limited resources is overwhelming. The primary burden of care for people with HIV/AIDS falls on the family. The families of the poor women of color who constitute the majority of women with AIDS in the United States have been devastated by the needs of their kin. Many of these families are headed by single mothers who have just finished caring for their own children when they take on the care of their sick daughters and often equally sick grandchildren (Simpson and Williams 1993). In addition to physical care and emotional support, they may have to battle with government and social service agencies to become legal foster parents, but if they care for their grandchildren informally, they lose out on benefits.

"AIDS Is Everyone's Trojan Horse"[28]

It is difficult to overestimate the immense and expansive social changes that have occurred in the wake of the first AIDS diagnosis. AIDS has changed ideas about sexual behavior, and not in ways predicted originally. Abstinence, monogamy, and condoms may have been the official recommendations, but innovative sexual practices in all kinds of couplings and social settings have also been the response to the search for "safer sex"

(Altman 1993). New sexual vocabularies ("serodiscordant couple"), sexual techniques (erotic massage), and protective devices ("dental dams"—mouth screens for oral sex) have been invented. Education programs for teenagers talk about the pleasures of nonpenetrative sexual expression that does not involve the exchange of body fluids, dubbed "outercourse" (Genuis and Genuis 1996). Some of these practices include phone sex, sharing sexual fantasies, and mutual masturbation. AIDS has also changed the relationships of people in the injecting drug communities as well as modifying social and public health policies aimed at them. Mothers, generally thought to be comforting, nurturing, and protecting, are potentially diseased vectors to the fetus and infants, who need drug protection in the womb.

AIDS also teaches us that neither men nor women are homogeneous and contrasting groups. The epidemiological statistics demonstrate that the disproportionate burden of AIDS has been on men and women of color, and more specifically, poor people in developing nations. But since women in these countries and in Western societies often have few economic resources, little social and political power, and carry the burden of family responsibilities, we can say that all the problems of AIDS have fallen most heavily on them.

Issues of gender justice, such as reconstructing the meaning of motherhood and social expectations of procreation and breastfeeding, access to information, freedom from sexual violence, and availability of prevention devices and cheap medicines, have different impacts on women throughout the world. Westernized heterosexual and bisexual women may have experienced the heady days of sexual liberation, when the pill and other woman-controlled means of contraception could be relied on to prevent pregnancy, but these days are gone, because these contraceptive devices do not protect against HIV infection. They never did protect against many other sexually transmitted diseases, but these were, for a while, curable.[29] Many lesbians can no longer hide behind the notion that they are safe, if their practices are more varied than their sexual identity may imply. Of course, women have never felt as invulnerable as heterosexual men have, because there is always the threat of rape, but for a short while, some women of privilege could be sexually adventurous without fear.

Some men now think about their bodies the way women do—as vulnerable and penetrable. Samuel Delany, in a piece about homosexuals' risk of AIDS, includes a comment from "a concerned and sensitive heterosexual woman friend: . . . 'AIDS has now put gay men in the position that straight women have always been in with sex: any unprotected sexual encounter now always carries with it the possibility of life or death'" (1991, 29). Some heterosexual men have HIV tests as "a way of re-establishing the integrity of the fragmented and penetrated body, the 'body besieged' in an age in which there are manifold anxieties concerning the purity of bodily fluids and the strength and resilience of one's immune system to fight invasion of viruses such as HIV" (Lupton et al. 1995, 104).

The competing messages of responsibility and powerlessness play out in the resurgence of HIV transmission in the very population that was so devastated by AIDS deaths and so politically active in getting drug research funded—young, gay men. Their growing casualness about condom use and other risky sexual behavior is matched by that of heterosexual adolescents. These young men and women know the "good" drug story—AIDS no longer equals death; you can take the drugs as a "morning after" prevention of infection. The ugly side is ancient history or happening on the other side of the world:

> Only a few years ago, gaunt men in wheelchairs haunted the streets of San Francisco's Castro District. The dark blotches of Karposi's sarcoma, a cancer linked to AIDS, flowered on cheeks and on forearms. Funeral homes struggled to meet the demand for their services. With the advent of drugs that prolong lives, though no one knows for how long, those daily horrors have faded. Instead, there are men tied to endless pill-taking regimens, who may suffer debilitating, occasionally fatal, side effects. But they look healthy, and they have returned to offices, gyms, restaurants and bars, restored to full—and fully sexual—lives. And as the obituaries have slowed, the balancing of safety and danger that is a theme in every life has shifted. (Goode 2001, 36)

In the new imagery, men's and women's bodies are not just passive recipients to be acted on; they are "both objects and agents of practice" (Connell 1995, 61). Socialized bodies, through sexual behavior and injected drug use, spread AIDS, and the people who "own" those bodies have been morally blamed and stigmatized for their risky behavior (Lupton 1993). But the body-social link is more complex—viruses become part of the body, living in it for years, sometimes without the "owner" knowing it, in benignly symbiotic or malignantly parasitic relationships.

AIDS as the most dreaded disease has replaced cancer, just the way cancer replaced tuberculosis, and tuberculosis replaced leprosy (Sontag 1989). Disease is not an invasion by a foreign element but part of a feedback loop system. The behavior of the social self who, through daily actions, interacts with other bodies and social selves, continuously reconstructs the body, which then acts on the social self. Through practices that change bodies, "more than individual lives are formed: a social world is formed" (Connell 1995: 64). It is this transformation of our social worlds by AIDS that will always be with us.

Summary

Biologically, AIDS is a disease transmitted through the exchange of infected bodily fluids. Socially, AIDS is a disease that is transmitted through social relationships. If one partner is HIV-positive, the other partner can be infected through their sexual couplings. Injection drug-using friends, family members, and lovers who exchange works or needles run the risk of transmitting HIV. HIV-positive mothers may expose their fetuses and infants to HIV through childbirth and breast feeding, turning normal mothering into a risky endeavor. A population that ended up almost completely HIV-infected are hemophiliacs, who were given contaminated blood transfusions in many countries even after there were good methods of sterilizing donated blood. Since the blood transfusions kept them alive and well through adolescence, many of them married and passed the virus to their partners and children before it was discovered that they were HIV-positive.

The premise of this book has been that all diseases are intertwined with social processes: Different social statuses put people at different risks and vary their access to health care. AIDS is a prime example. Another premise has been that the social status of those who are ill is less an effect of their individual behavior than of their society's evaluation of them as people. With AIDS, hemophiliacs and their wives are heroic victims of their governments' refusal to purify the blood hemophiliacs used to stay alive; injection drug users and their wives are stigmatized as perpetrators of their own physical decline, even though a supply of free, clean needles by governments would be a cheap way to prevent transmission of the HIV virus.

In AIDS, as in other diseases, epidemiological data collection has been hampered by outmoded categories of risk groups that concentrate on individual characteristics and neglect the patterns of transmission and prevention in local community networks and peer groups. In the past twenty years, tracking has been of supposed dangerous cases—gay men, prostitutes, intravenous drug users—neglecting middle-class and poor heterosexual men and women and entire populations of developing countries. Governments were slow to finance research and low-cost treatment and prevention programs when the populations at risk were poor people of color or women of any racial group and class, but they prioritized finding a cure when HIV infection threatened middle- and upper-class heterosexual men. The intense pressure of social activists unrelentingly attacked government agencies, medical systems, and drug companies, bringing about some lessening of the foot-dragging and profit-driven behavior of these powerful institutions.

Health care in Westernized countries, as we have seen, is oriented to cure, not prevention; to individual treatment of specific pathologies as they occur, not to strengthening physical, emotional, and social capacities for living with a chronic or recurrent disease. People with AIDS in particular have needed, and not always obtained, such holistic care. The social supports that have mitigated the ravages of AIDS have been supplied by their families, lovers, friends, and community-organized services, not by the medical or social welfare system. In non-Westernized countries, where much of the population suffers from malnutrition and other infections, AIDS is an epidemic like the medieval Black Death in Europe—a plague that kills a substantial proportion of young adults. Whole generations have died in some communities.

Certainly, the scientific research effort has paid off—the HIV virus was discovered, and more and more of its immune cell-binding properties have been revealed, including genetic and drug protectors. But much less money and time has been spent on the social aspects of transmission and health care. In retrospect, it seems astounding that no one tried to prevent the inevitable spread to injection drug users by contaminated needles, given the scrupulous disposal of needles in medical settings. The assumption that women could not get AIDS unless they were prostitutes is attributable to the moral contrast of categories of people (gay men vs. heterosexual men; prostitute women vs. respectable women), an astonishingly naive misunderstanding of sexual behavior and sexual practices. Equally naive has been the assumption that education in safe sex and condom use would halt the spread of AIDS in *any* population. Again, the gender dynamics of relationships were ignored, as well as the cultural meanings of condoms and social meanings of love and trust.

The AIDS epidemic is talked of as "exceptional," and has been treated as a "special case" in public health (Scheper-Hughes 1994). But in actuality, AIDS is not an exception—the problems of this epidemic are the problems of Western and non-Western health care systems writ large, with the same issues of gender, racial, ethnic, and class disadvantage that have been discussed throughout this book.

AIDS has been different from other epidemics in one major respect: Despite dire predictions of quarantine and other means of social control of those who test HIV-positive, it has not, at least in democracies, resulted in mandatory testing, increased government surveillance, or loss of civil liberties. The downside of this policy of voluntary action is that the onus for protection is placed on the individual, who must be aware of risks and suspicious of sexual partners and constantly negotiate self-protection. Into this negotiation go differences in power and privileges, and a gender analysis tells us who usually wins and who usually loses. As Scheper-Hughes says, "Until all people—women and children in particular—share equal rights in social and sexual citizenship, an AIDS program built exclusively on individual rights to bodily autonomy and privacy cannot possibly represent the needs of groups who have been historically excluded from these" (1994, 1002).

The "strong and humane public health system" she calls for needs to be matched by a medical system sensitive to gender dynamics and gender politics. At the same time, individuals do have to know how to protect their own health *and* the health of those in their intimate networks *and* the health of their children, but they should not be blamed if their immune systems are so weakened by a virus and social and environmental bodily assaults that they ultimately break down. The intricate interplay of individual freedom and institutional protections, of medical care and social needs, of attention to special cases and even-handed distribution of personal and societal resources—these ambiguities and complexities are the heart of the social construction of AIDS and, indeed, of all illnesses.

NOTES

1. Tracking by the U.S. Centers for Disease Control (CDC) began in 1981, but it took years before the persistent medical reports of a strange pneumonia and a rare cancer among young, gay men got a response from the government (Shilts 1987).

2. Almost all the hemophiliacs who were infused with blood-clotting factors between the mid-1970s and the mid-1980s are HIV-positive (Kolata 1991). Most of the HIV-positive hemophiliac adults are married men, and a high percentage of their wives are also infected (Patton 1994, 59–65).

3. A double copy of the gene protects against infection; a single copy seems to delay the development of AIDS symptoms by five to ten years.

4. "Women and HIV / AIDS," Fact Sheet, 2001. Kaiser Family Foundation Web site.

5. On issues in the constructionist perspective on AIDS, see Levine 1992 and Treichler 1992, 1999.

6. The first reports of opportunistic infections were of pneumocystis carinii pneumonia and Karposi's sarcoma, which produce lesions in the skin, mucous membranes, and internal organs. They were rarely seen by American physicians before the late 1970s. There are now more than thirty different conditions that can proliferate when immune systems are weakened by HIV.

7. "AIDS Epidemic Update," December 2001. UNAIDS Web site.

8. See note 4.

9. For early reports, see Masur et al. 1992 and Wallace et al. 1983. On the slow response of the medical profession, see Corea 1992 and Patton 1994. For recent issues, see Goldstein and Manlowe 1997.

10. "The Status and Trends of the HIV/AIDS Epidemic in the World, 2000." U.S. Census Bureau Web site.

11. Since there is a double economy of sex and drugs, the CDC now has a category, "people who trade sex for drugs or money" (Patton 1994, 56).

12. Epidemics also stabilize when the population at risk is "saturated"—there are few uninfected people (Bloor 1995, 31–32).

13. The interpretation of statistics can be confusing and appear contradictory. In recent years U.S. statistics have revealed that while the incidence rate (number of new cases) of HIV/AIDS has decreased in certain communities, the prevalence rate (number of existing cases) has increased. That is because people are now living longer with HIV/AIDS, thanks to combination drug therapy, so the total number of cases increases as new cases are added to existing cases.

14. "Innovative Approaches to HIV Prevention: Selected Case Studies." 2000. UNAIDS Web site.

15. U.S. Department of Justice Web site, 2000.

16. "HIV and AIDS in the Americas: An Epidemic with Many Faces." 2000. UNAIDS Web site.

17. For a discussion of risk reduction of HIV and sexually transmitted diseases with incarcerated women, see Hogben and St. Lawrence 2000.

18. The Female Health Company and UNAIDS have negotiated a lower price to launch a promotional campaign in several developing nations.

19. For discussions of power, culture, and women's relationships in HIV transmission and postinfection survival, see Amaro and Raj 2000, Jenkins 2000, and Reid 2000.

20. Also see Browne and Minichiello 1996, Kelly 1995b, and Lear 1995.

21. "Trends in the HIV and AIDS Epidemic, 1998." CDC Web site.

22. "Key Findings from CDC: HIV/AIDS Update 2001." CDC Web site.

23. UNAIDS estimates 13.2 million orphans since the beginning of the epidemic. "Report on Global HIV/AIDS Epidemic: AIDS Epidemic Update Report." 2000. UNAIDS Web site.

24. See note 23.

25. On the contradictions of leaving women out of the original AZT trials because the drug might do fetal damage and then designing a trial to ascertain how protective of fetuses AZT is, see Corea 1992, 204–6.

26. Women knowingly have children with higher rates of potentially fatal inheritable diseases.

27. "Access to Drugs: UNAIDS Technical Update." 1998. UNAIDS Web site. A *New York Times* series on South Africa was called "Death and Denial" (November 25–30, 2001).

28. Sontag 1989: 168.

29. Gonorrhea soon became resistant to penicillin; genital and oral herpes viruses are never completely eradicated. These and other sexually transmitted diseases have become almost incurable opportunistic infections in women with AIDS.

CHAPTER 8

Healing Social Bodies in Social Worlds: Feminist Health Care

> In these exchanges the social certainly interrupts and interpenetrates the medical. Whether medical or social topics are being discussed, social/ ideological assumptions are clearly embedded in the discourse. (Fisher 1995, 59)

We have argued in this book that across the globe the experiences of health, disability, and illness are socially constructed. Bodies, physiology, and genetics vary from individual to individual, and also from group to group. Sex categories are one set of groupings, and others are age cohorts and racial ethnic clusters. Although these groups seem to be defined by physiological factors, social factors are embedded in them. Sex categories invoke gender statuses, with all the weight of social expectations, opportunities, and limitations. Age categories are as much social as physiological—the formal status of "senior" at age sixty-five brings social privileges in certain countries that come with physical markers (menopause, white hair). Racial ethnic genetic variations, such as propensity to sickle-cell anemia or cystic fibrosis, have social as well as physical effects. The illness symptoms are experienced in the body, but chronic illness becomes a social role. Where you live has many social and physical effects—availability of clean water or any water at all, access to food and cultural varieties of diet, pressures to bear children, not bear them, bear many, abort those of one sex. In short, there is no aspect of human life that is not at one and the same time physical, environmental, and social.

Health, illness, and disability are particularly multiple—experienced by individuals in bodies, defined by experts and authorities, and significantly influenced by economic resources, nutrition, type of work done, family responsibilities, and socioemotional supports. These social factors cluster in systems of expectations and practices legitimated by norms and values, which sociologists call *institutions*—the economy, the family, the medical system, the gender order. In modern society, *organizations*, such as hospitals, link individuals to institutions (and institutions to each other). A patient in a hospital in the United States may be getting sick pay from a job and medical insurance from a health care agency, linking the economic and medical systems. The patient is also a family member, and his or her relationships with partner, children, siblings, and parents intertwine the medical system with the family as a social institution.

What this book has stressed is that health, illness, and disability are experienced through gender norms, social class privileges and disadvantages, and racial ethnic cultures. Medical researchers use many physical, psychological, and social variables in trying to explain health behavior—risk behavior in HIV transmission, for instance. They frequently come up with mixed outcomes and few clear patterns on the individual or dyadic level. But when sociologists have used *social system* data (class, racial and ethnic group, sexual and gender status) to explain the spread of AIDS, the patterns are much clearer. Those most disadvantaged have a higher risk of HIV infection, and they are, throughout the world, poor women and men of color. Social epidemiological data is better explained by social system factors than by individual behavior.

Most social researchers concentrate on these social system, organizational, and interactive effects, and include the social and environmental factors that affect physiological functioning, such as pollution and smoking. Biomedical research, in contrast, puts much less emphasis on social factors. Because the knowledge base of modern medicine is rooted in the sciences (biology, biochemistry, physiology, endocrinology, and so on), the social and environmental aspects of disease and the experience of illness are given less attention in medical training and practice. The body is dissected in medical school, and its functions and dysfunctions are memorized. But in order to understand the complexities of illness as a social experience, you cannot look only at the patient's body. Even adding psychological characteristics is not enough. Illness takes place within a web of interaction that ties together the person concerned, family, friends, coworkers, health care professionals, medical bureaucracies, the physical setting, technology, government policies and politics, economics, values, knowledge, and beliefs.

Social Contingencies of Health Care Delivery

The feminist perspective on health care argues that the social factors that construct health and illness should be an integral part of medical knowledge and medical practice. It also argues that the patient's perspective and a caring ethic should be integrated into treatment regimens. This means that the patient's account of his or her illness is attended to seriously and that the patient is given complete information in an understandable way and encouraged to take responsibility for all decisions.

The concept of *social interaction* is particularly applicable to encounters between patients and health care professionals. Compare a health provider's likely response to a man and a woman, both heterosexual, African-American, middle-class, fifty-year-old divorced bank managers with cardiovascular symptoms. The man's irregular heartbeat and fainting spells would probably elicit a battery of tests and specific treatment; the woman's identical symptoms would probably elicit a prescription for tranquilizers for emotional stress. We could similarly compare the experiences in an infertility clinic of a woman and man who are both heterosexual, White, working-class, twenty-three-year-old married post office clerks with infertility due to adolescent bouts of gonorrhea. The woman may find that her sexual past creates skepticism about her mothering capabilities in the eyes of the staff of the infertility clinic, but the same staff will most probably urge his partner to undergo *in vitro* fertilization so he might have a biological child. In all these cases, the outcome would probably be modified by varying the gender and racial ethnic group of the health care provider, and their similarity to or difference from the patient.

Within the United States, the demographics of the medical profession are changing, and physicians are likely to be mostly women in the near future, and of diverse racial and ethnic groups. One reason for the influx of women is that the authority of doctors has been eroded and their income has gone down with more and more medical care under the jurisdiction of governments or large insurance companies. At the same time, patients' rights movements have diminished physicians' professional prestige. As a result, fewer men are going into medicine, leaving room for more women, who are fast becoming the majority of doctors in every country with a Western medical system. Some of these women physicians are challenging medicine's biology-based perspective, as are men physicians with a holistic perspective on medical care. Medical school curricula and training, however, are still focused on individual bodies and their pathologies, with a smattering of courses in public health, environmental and occupational diseases, nutrition, stress, and family medicine.

Much medical care is delivered by nonphysician personnel, especially nurses, who are still mostly women. Their numbers have not made the medical profession as a whole woman-dominated in practices and values because the professional hierarchy puts physicians at the top of the authority chain. Physicians' power to define the medical encounter comes from their authority as experts in biomedical science and technology. Despite nursing's ethic of care and concern for the patient, in technology-based biomedicine, nurses are more often busy with the mechanics and instrumentalities of patient care than with dispensing TLC. Listening to the patient's emotional and social problems is relegated to nurses' aides and other personnel even further down the professional hierarchy, who don't get paid to listen but to do physical care. Even patients who recover at home get less and less TLC. They are discharged early with more complicated treatment routines and physical care, such as wound dressings and injections, to be administered in the home. The stress of the situation makes it hard for the home caregiver to have time or energy for the sick person's emotional needs.

Unfortunately, payment and profit are driving much of the way health care is provided by Western medicine today. Everything in health care is governed by insurers' or government rules about what can or cannot be done, who does it, and for how long. Managed care and national health services are organized to cut costs to meet budgetary or profit bottom lines, not to provide quality, comprehensive services.

Women's and Men's Health Movements

One source of change from within the medical profession has been the focus on women's health coming from organizations and journals of women physicians. They have built on the feminist perspective that illness and cure are social as well as individual. Some feminist physicians have recommended the development of a specialty in women's health that is not "a reproductive surgical specialty" but rather treats women "as whole human beings with minds, bodies, and spirits—separate and distinct from men's—and worthy of an equal investment in scientific study, clinical education, and medical services" (Johnson and Hoffman 1994, 36–37). This specialty would be interdisciplinary, treating lung and colon cancer as well as ovarian cancer, domestic violence and rape as well as infertility. There have been proposals for similar nurse practitioner programs to provide primary health care addressed to women's needs (Cohen et al. 1994). A women's health medical and nursing specialty would be similar to gerontology, adolescent medicine, and pediatrics, which serve the special physical, psychological, and social problems of people of different ages.

An alternative approach to women's health care is to create expert knowledge that could be taught to family practitioners and other primary care physicians and incorporated into medical and nursing school curricula and textbooks. In 1990, under the auspices of the American Medical Women's Association, a group of women representing medical societies and women's health consumer organizations drafted a core curriculum "to improve and integrate the care of women patients, heighten physicians' awareness of the psychosocial aspects of women's treatment, improve the physician-patient partnership, and increase the physicians' understanding of the differences and unique qualities of women's health" (Wallis 1994, 21). The curriculum is divided into five life-phase modules (early years, young adult, midlife, mature years, advanced years), and covers nine content areas: sexuality and reproduction, women and society, health maintenance and wellness, violence and abuse, mental health and substance abuse, transition and changes, patient-physician partnership, normal female physiology, and diagnosis and management of conditions common to the five age groups. Michelle Harrison, who does not favor a separate women's health specialty because she feels that all of medicine and health care should address the needs of women, nevertheless suggests a master's degree in women's health to provide experts who could develop programs, design research, and teach a variety of health care personnel (1994).

The social contexts of men's illnesses have become a similar focus of an international men's health movement, with its own organizations, Web sites, journals, and conferences (Baker 2001). About ten years old, this movement takes the feminist critique of Western biomedical perspectives, which argued for greater attention to social and environmental causes of illness, and applies them to men's health.[1] As Alice Dan says in her introduction to *Reframing Women's Health*, "Why should context be any more significant for women than for men? Men's lives are also lived within a context" (1994, xv). The normative assumptions about health and illness may be built on men's lives and minimize women's special needs, but views of "normality" also ignore the health care needs of working-class men, men of color, and bisexuals and homosexuals.

The physicians working with the men's health movement recognize that just as women's overall social status makes them vulnerable to illnesses of poverty and to procreative and sexual coercion, so does men's social status put them at risk for traumas, drug and alcohol abuse, homicide, and suicide. Given the gender-segregated structure of work, men's jobs are sometimes very hazardous. Norms of masculinity shape their responses to traumas—boys are taught to "play through pain" and to deny or ignore illness symptoms (Moynihan 1998). Men in middle management suffer the stress of responsibility with too little authority and little encouragement to talk about their feelings. Poor men, who are most likely to be suffering from multiple physical problems, usually have the most difficulty in obtaining comprehensive care.

Just as the feminist health movement called for greater attention to gender privileges and inequities in researching women's illnesses and health care for women, the men's health movement uses these concepts in looking at the particular risks to men's health of their work, sexual behavior, eating patterns, smoking, drinking, and drug use. Beyond individual risk-taking, an even more important focus of the men's health movement are social and cultural factors that affect men's health—racism, masculine bravado, encouragement of violence, and the drive to make money and rise in one's career (Riska 2002). The feminist health movement strengthened women's assertiveness in getting proper diagnoses and health care compatible with their social needs. The men's health movement is also encouraging men to attend to their physical and emotional health, to express their needs and not bury them under a façade of masculine stoicism (and put themselves in an early grave).

When the women's health movement began in the 1970s, it was extremely critical of Western medicine's masculine bias and neglect of the social context of individual illnesses. Feminist criticism at the time called for reformation of the whole health care system—increasing the autonomy of the woman patient and the authority of nonphysician women health care providers, exploration of alternative modes of treatment beyond drugs and surgery, and putting women's bodies and life-cycles in the forefront of care. The men's health movement, as well as the patient's rights movement, has inherited the changes feminist critiques helped bring to Western health care systems. Today, all patients are encouraged to become "experts" in their own health care. Much care is provided by non-MD professionals, men as well as women. Alternative medicine (herbal drugs, nutrition, meditation, acupuncture) are part of standard care.

The emphasis the men's health movement places on individual responsibility for one's health and the cooperation of the layperson and health care providers reflects similar recommendations by the women's health movement today. Both, however, are still critical of the uneven attention given by the medical profession and by governments to the environment, preventive medicine, and public health issues. Pharmaceutical and biotechnological short-term solutions receive much more funding and critical attention than air and water pollution, unhealthy food additives, and genetic modification of foods and fetuses.

Participatory Medical Encounters

The social structure of health care and the social contingencies of illness are the "surround" for individual experiences. The face-to-face interaction with the medical system for patients is with health care providers. The ideal for patient-provider interactions is for patients to participate as equals in the decisions about their care. Providers supply expert knowledge of the body and its functionings, and their experience with the likely course of chronic and acute illnesses under different treatment regimens. Patients bring expert knowledge of their own body and its functioning, their illness history, and their reactions to drugs, surgeries, and other treatments they have undergone. If patients are going to be full participants in medical encounters, they must be given time to describe the context of a particular illness episode, as well as its time span (Candib 1988). In turn, the health care professional must "accept as valid another person's experience in shaping his or her way of looking at the world," and in "listening actively," indicate that she or he respects the patient's interpretation of events surrounding the illness (p. 135).

Participatory medical encounters call for unhurried professionals and patients skilled in conveying the significant details of their physical problem and its social context. All the accounts of medical encounters show, when asked, "What's wrong?" patients do say what's bothering them and why it is of concern to them, how long the problem has been going on, and, if given the chance, narrate its history. Very often, it is not lack of time to listen that's the difficulty, it's that physicians, in particular, hear only what *they* think is important to know—the cues for the physical, body-located source of the "abnormality." They cut off the patient's story because they rarely credit social factors, such as losing a job, as equally valid evidence for someone getting sick or having a recurrence of chronic symptoms. However, they bring social factors back in when they prescribe treatments and other remedies, because they are asking the patient to act in ways that the physician thinks best.

Sue Fisher points out that although caring is the hallmark of nursing, and nurse-practitioners pride themselves on probing for the social aspects of a patient's symptoms, they, too, are likely to try to impose their definition of the situation as the solution to the patient's overall difficulties (1995). Thus, in a case she analyzes, the nurse-practitioner discusses divorce with a patient whose marital difficulties have made her ill, but the patient resists that solution. Since nurse-patient encounters are less asymmetrical in authority and power than those between doctors and patients (especially when the doctor is a man and the patient a woman), there is more room for "bargaining." In Fisher's case, the compromise suggested by the patient and validated by the nurse-practitioner is to go out more with her friends and take up running again.

There is no doubt that patients have to struggle to make themselves heard in most medical encounters, and that a more open "ear" on the part of practitioners would help reveal the "multilayered, complex, and fluid" aspects of illnesses (Fisher 1994, 326). But professionals and patients have social identities and viewpoints that may conflict, and the given in any *medical* setting is that the professional has the authority, power, prestige, and greater knowledge. A feminist practice puts the burden of change on the professional, not the patient. It is up to the professional to make sure that he or she hears the patient's description of both the physical symptoms and the social context, that the patient understands the physiological aspects of the problem and the alternatives for treatment (and nontreatment, too), and that the patient make the decisions (not just agree to them) and be given support and referrals even if the professional doesn't agree with the patient's decisions.

Being a Patient

A project that has been useful in helping students understand the multiple impacts of patients' social characteristics on encounters with the health care system analyzes the experience of being a patient. Students use their own experiences or interview someone they know well. These questions cover the gamut of factors that go into the social construction of an illness experience:

1. What is your age, gender, ethnicity, racial group, religion, education, occupation, and sexual orientation? What is your relationship status;

how many children or adults are you responsible for; who do you live with? Do you have health insurance?

2. What were the initial stages of a new illness or an acute episode of a chronic illness? What were the symptoms? How did you interpret them? What was the input of family, friends, coworkers, and other nonprofessionals? What self-medication did you use? Did you remember a TV or newspaper advertisement for a medicine that would apply to your case? Did you go on the Internet to get information? At what point and why did you consult a health care professional, in person or by phone? What were your choices? What kind of professional did you choose? Why did you choose this professional?

3. What was this professional's interpretation of the symptoms? What kinds of tests or examinations did you have? Did you see any other professionals before a diagnosis was made? What was the diagnosis? Who made the diagnosis? Did you help make the diagnosis? Did you agree with the diagnosis? What were the recommendations for treatment? Did you think you could do what the professional said you had to do to get better? Did you do them?

4. Describe what happened in one particular encounter in this illness. What was the setting—e.g., office, clinic, hospital emergency room? Who, besides you, was present (which health care workers, family members)? What were the occupational status and the social characteristics (approximate age, gender, racial or ethnic group, etc.) of the health care workers present? What exactly went on? How was the work divided? Were there areas of conflict or argument? What were they? How were they resolved? How did you feel (satisfied, angry, upset) during and after this encounter? Did you have to get clearance from your health insurer for this visit? How did you pay for this visit? For the medication you were prescribed?

5. How did (or does) the illness impact on your family and work obligations? Who took care of you? Were they compensated? Did you return to normal functioning or were your occupational and familial status changed by the illness? In what ways did they change?

As you can see, a patient's whole social world is involved in a major illness, and a whole professional world influences one health care encounter. Although the patient may challenge, resist, and counteract, the assumptions that prevail are likely to be those of the health care professional, especially if she or he is a physician. One way of equalizing the power differential somewhat is for lay people to become more knowledge-able about medicine and science in general and about any serious illness they may have. Thanks to the consumer movement and the feminist move-ment, lay people have become more aware of tests, medications, the causes of different illnesses, treatment alternatives, and likely outcomes. Informa-tion about illnesses and treatments are available on the net for those with access to computers.

However, what we learn in the mass media and on the internet has been filtered through several editing processes. First, research projects must be funded by either a federal agency, such as the National Institutes of Health, or a pharmaceutical company with self-interest in the outcome of a clini- cal trial. Not all illnesses are deemed either critical or profitable enough to be funded, and there is limited scientific knowledge about some conditions that make it impossible for someone to live a normal life but are not con-sidered physically life-threatening, such as chronic pain or chronic fatigue.

Data produced by researchers in laboratories and clinical trials become part of scientific communications, most desirably within the most presti-gious journals or at large international conferences. Funding agencies, laboratories, research teams, and government agencies use press confer-ences and press releases to call attention to noteworthy projects and their results. Journalists use only the most newsworthy items for their articles in mass media newspapers and magazines and in information newsletters on the Internet. At this point, much of the scientific content of the original research agenda is summarized in dramatic and positive language. By the time it gets to TV, much of the information is reduced to a sound bite that can sometimes be misleading and is almost always an upbeat presentation of scientific research and new drugs and surgical procedures. In assessing such information, it helps to remember that "producers and those with whom they create knowledge are always located somewhere, and that somewhere is always imbedded in cultural specifics that shape how knowledges are produced and disseminated" (Olesen and Clarke 1999, 356).

Making Changes

Participatory models in health care created by feminists have led to sig-nificant changes. In order to demonstrate the power and potential of social transformation in health care, we will describe two examples of revision-ist feminist health care: the first, in our understanding of human genital anatomy, and the second, in access to treatment and information about breast cancer.

Human anatomical textbooks have historically been based on dissections of male bodies (Moore and Clarke 2001). One of the few places where women and girls could see what female bodies look like and how they function have been the many international editions of *Our Bodies, Ourselves*. However, depictions of genitalia in most other sites have not given women's and men's anatomies equal space and variety. Using feminist critiques of standard anatomical representations, the Federation of Feminist Women's Health Centers commissioned and published a radically different anatomy of women's bodies, with a complete redefinition of the clitoris. *A New View of a Woman's Body*[2] is partially based on interviews with women and includes several color photographs of different women's genital anatomy. These images and descriptions show a wide range of genital variation and provide deeper understanding of their sexual, and not exclusively reproductive, function. Similarly, feminist poet and essayist Audre Lorde (1980) has explored the political implications of prosthetic breasts, arguing that hiding women's pain and suffering disguises the widespread nature of breast cancer and places too much emphasis on "normal" femininity.[3]

From the micropolitical issues of reconstructing "feminine" bodies to the macropolitical concerns of environmental clean-up of toxins, breast cancer activism provides multiple examples of the power of participatory feminist organizing in health care. Between 1990 and 1993, breast cancer activism became a significant political movement. Through the feminist organizing of heterogeneous groups of women, diagnosis, treatment, and clinical trials of breast cancer began to receive extensive media attention. Breast cancer activists have used a wide spectrum of approaches, from corporate sponsorship and grassroots community organizing, to create new partnerships, collaborations, research funding opportunities, and avenues for access to quality care. Survivors of breast cancer have become major players in public policy, science, industry, and advocacy about the disease.

Breast cancer activism has included and ignited other health care activism. Prostate cancer activism has used breast cancer activism's models for popularizing self-examinations and garnering financial support for research. For example, a series of community-based running events similar to the Susan G. Komen Foundation's "Race for the Cure," premiered in 1998 in New York City's Central Park as part of National Prostate Cancer Awareness Week.

These examples of collaborations of laypeople and professionals in making changes show that it is possible to change thinking and practices and, in the process, produce scientific knowledge that is rooted in the social contexts of people's lives.

Summary

Humans differ genetically, hormonally, physiologically, environmentally, and socially from prenatal development to death, and much research time and effort have gone into trying to separate out causal factors of illnesses and pathologies. From a biomedical perspective, isolation of the prime cause (a bacterium, virus, gene or genetic mutation, a hormone or its lack, an element of diet, smoking, and so on) is the ideal, modeled after the nineteenth-century discovery that specific "germs" cause specific diseases. But after a century that has seen the design of antibacterials, antivirals, insulin, vitamins, and vaccines to handle diseases caused by specific deficiencies or invaders, we now face chronic disorders of the cardiovascular, respiratory, and immune systems. These diseases are particularly responsive to social factors, such as the way we live and work, and to the environment, which can trigger genetic predispositions.

The biosocial interaction, we now know, is a feedback loop. Bodies affect social life, and social life affects bodies. What bodies are doesn't dictate behavior; people with relationships and social ties and social statuses decide how their bodies should act. Yet rather than look for the skills, environments, and networks for altering risky behavior, we often expect that there will be a medical technology for dealing with the consequences of our actions—cures for sexually transmitted diseases, orthopedic surgery for sports traumas. Medical technology has provided those with access to it with many valuable treatments, but as people live longer, the illnesses they incur are more likely to be chronic. Management of these long-term conditions involves social resources as well as medicines and surgeries.

In order to understand the incidence, prevalence, and transmission of chronic or acute diseases, researchers have had to consider a population's body typologies and genetic pool, social practices that affect bodies directly (what people eat, drink, smoke), social environments (where people live, the work they do), social and sexual networks that influence individual behavior and provide emotional supports, and access to health care resources, technology, and knowledge. Similarly, a context-based health practice looks at the whole life of an individual to understand the causes and effects of a set of symptoms and to decide on the most productive course of treatment and adaptation to diminished capabilities.

Illnesses and disabilities are deeply embedded in the *social* order. The expert knowledge for comprehensive health care therefore has to start with *social worlds* and work back from social processes to their impact on bodies. In practice, that knowledge can be applied to particular patients, working back and forth from their social worlds to their socially constituted bodies. The knowledge of different social worlds should not be confined to practitioners from those worlds—we are not suggesting that only practitioners who share all of a patient's social characteristics can treat that patient. What is more important is that practitioners from different social worlds learn about health and illness through the prism of the social, which refracts the supposedly universal human body and its functions and dysfunctions into diverse and various *social bodies*.

The model of health care explored in this chapter is based on feminist principles: universal access to quality care, attention to the whole life of the patient, participatory diagnoses and treatment decisions, and professional support for the patient to carry out these joint decisions. One of the most profound lessons to be gained from exploring health and illness as social constructions is in understanding your own role in the production of the social meaning of your body and your experiences of health and illness. As potential patients and caregivers, we each have an investment in the ways in which health and illness are constructed. We are not merely passive receptacles of diagnoses and treatment options; we are also participants in the creation of health care. We have continually examined how individuals are constrained by their social environments. Simultaneously, we implore readers to view themselves as full of potential for resistance to and transformation of these very social environments.

NOTES

1. For overviews of feminist perspectives on men's health, see Sabo and Gordon 1993 and Doyal 2001.

2. Written and published by the Federation of Feminist Women's Health Centers West, Hollywood, Calif., 1981, illustrated by Suzann Gage.

3. Also see Kasper (1995).

REFERENCES

Abbreviations:
BMJ – British Medical Journal
Differences – Differences: A Journal of Feminist Cultural Studies
JAMA – Journal of the American Medical Association
JAMWA – Journal of the American Medical Women's Association
JWH – Journal of Women's Health, as of 1999 Journal of Women's Health and Gender–Based Medicine
NYT –The New York Times
Signs – Signs: Journal of Women in Culture and Society

AADS (American Association of Dental Schools) 1997. "Trends in Dental Education and Faculty." Washington, D.C.: AADS.

AAP (American Academy of Pediatrics). 1999. "Circumcision Policy Statement." *Pediatrics* 103: 686–93.

Abbey, A., F. M. Andrews, and J. L. Halman. 1991. "Gender's Role in Responses to Infertility." *Psychology of Women Quarterly* 15: 295–316.

Abimiku, A. G., and R. C. Gallo. 1995. "HIV: Basic Virology and Pathophysiology." Pp.13–31 in *HIV Infection in Women*, edited by H. Minkoff, J. A. DeHovitz, and A. Duerr. New York: Raven Press.

Abplanalp, J. M. 1983."Premenstrual Syndrome: A Selective Review." *Women and Health* 8 (2,3): 107–23.

Abramsky, L., S. Hall, J. Levitan et al. 2001. "What Parents Are Told after Prenatal Diagnosis of a Sex Chromosome Abnormality: Interview and Questionnaire Study." *BMJ* 322: 463–66.

Abusharaf, R. M. 2001. "Virtuous Cuts: Female Genital Mutilation in an African Ontology." *Differences* 12(Spring): 112–40.

Agee, E. 2000. "Menopause and the Transmission of Women's Knowledge: African American and White Women's Perspectives." *Medical Anthropology Quarterly* 14: 73–95.

Ahmed, A., N. H. Mbibi, D. Dawam et al. 1999. "Complications of Traditional Male Circumcision." *Annals of Tropical Pediatrics: International Child Health* 19: 113–17.

Aldeeb Abu-Sahlieh, S. A. 1994. "To Mutilate in the Name of Jehovah or Allah: Legitimization of Male and Female Circumcision." *Medicine and Law* 13(7–8): 575–622.

Alonso, A. M. and M. T. Koreck. 1989. "Silences: 'Hispanics,' AIDS, and Sexual Practices." *Differences* 1(Winter): 101–24.

Altman, D. 1993. "AIDS and the Discourses of Sexuality." Pp. 32–48 in *Rethinking Sex: Social Theory and Sexuality Research*, edited by R. W. Connell and G. W. Dowsett. Philadelphia: Temple University Press.

Altman, L. 2001. "Study Reports Drug-Resistant Strains Have Increased to 14 Percent Among New HIV Cases." *NYT*, February 8.

151

————. 2000. "Promise and Peril of New Drugs for AIDS." *NYT,* February 8.

Amaro, H., and A. Raj. 2000. "On the Margin: Power and Women's HIV Risk Reduction Strategies. *Sex Roles* 42: 723–49.

Andersen, A. E., editor. 1990. *Males with Eating Disorders.* New York: Brunner/ Mazel.

Anderson, E. 1989. "Sex Codes and Family Life among Poor Inner-City Youths." *Annals of the American Academy of Political and Social Science* 501: 59–78.

Anonymous. 2001. "Osteoporosis Prevention, Diagnosis, and Therapy" *JAMA* 285: 785–95.

Anson, O., A. Levenson, and D. Y. Bonneh. 1990. "Gender and Health on the Kibbutz." *Sex Roles* 22: 213–35.

Applegate, J. S. and L. W. Kaye. 1993. "Male Elder Caregivers." Pp. 152–67 in *Doing "Women's Work": Men in Non-Traditional Occupations,* edited by C. L. Williams. Thousand Oaks, Calif.: Sage.

Araton, H. 2001. "A Champion Slips Away Unnoticed." *NYT,* August 30.

Asch, A., and M. Fine. 1988. "Introduction: Beyond Pedestals." Pp. 1–37 in *Women with Disabilities: Essays in Psychology, Culture, and Politics,* edited by M. Fine and A. Asch. Philadelphia: Temple University Press.

Asch, A., and L. H. Sacks. 1983. "Lives Without, Lives Within: Autobiographies of Blind Women and Men." *Journal of Visual Impairment and Blindness* 77: 242–47.

Ashley, J. A. 1976. *Hospitals, Paternalism, and the Role of the Nurse.* New York: Teachers College Press.

Avis, N. E., and S. M. McKinlay. 1995. "The Massachusetts Women's Health Study: An Epidemiological Investigation of the Menopause." *JAMWA* 50: 45–49, 63.

Avis, N. E., R. Stellano, S. Crawford et al. 2001. "Is There a Menopausal Syndrome? Menopausal Status and Symptoms across Racial/Ethnic Groups." *Social Science and Medicine* 52: 345–56.

Bailey, R., R. Muga, and R. Poulussen. 2000. "Trial Intervention Introducing Male Circumcision to Reduce HIV/STD Infections in Nyanza Province, Kenya: Baseline Results." Abstracts of the XIII International AIDS Conference, Durban, South Africa.

Baker, P. 2001. "The International Men's Health Movement." *BMJ* 323: 1014–15.

Barnett, E. A. 1988."*Le Edad Critica*: The Positive Experience of Menopause in a Small Peruvian Town." Pp. 40–54 in *Women and Health: Cross-Cultural Perspectives,* edited by P. Whelehan and contributors. Granby, Mass.: Bergin and Garvey.

Barr, K. E. M., M. P. Farrell, G. M. Barnes et al. 1993. "Race, Class, and Gender Differences in Substance Abuse: Evidence of Middle-Class/Underclass Polarization among Black Males." *Social Problems* 40: 314–27.

Barroso, C. 1994. "Building a New Specialization on Women's Health: An International Perspective." Pp. 93–101 in *Reframing Women's Health,* edited by A. J. Dan. Newbury Park, Calif.: Sage.

Bartman, B., and E. Moy. 1998. "Racial Differences in Estrogen Use among Middle-Aged and Older Women." *Women's Health Issues* 8: 32–44.

Bashir, L. Miller. 1997. "Female Genital Mutilation: Balancing Intolerance of the Practice with Tolerance of Culture." *JWH* 6: 11–14.

Bauer, G. R. and S. L. Welles. 2001. "Beyond Assumptions of Negligible Risk: Sexually Transmitted Diseases and Women Who Have Sex with Women." *American Journal of Public Health* 91: 1282–86.

Bayley, J. 1998. *Elegy for Iris.* New York: St. Martin's Press.

Bayne-Smith, M. 1996. *Race, Gender, and Health.* Newbury Park, Calif.: Sage.

Becker, G., and J. K. Jauregui. 1985. "The Invisible Isolation of Deaf Women: Its Effect on Social Awareness." Pp. 23–36 in *Women and Disability: The Double Handicap,* edited by M. J. Deegan and N. A. Brooks. New Brunswick, N.J.: Transaction Books.

Bell, S. E. 1990. "The Medicalization of Menopause." Pp. 43–63 in *The Meaning of Menopause: Historical, Medical, and Clinical Perspectives,* edited by R. Formanek. Hillsdale, N.J.: Analytic Press.

Ben-Tovim, D. I., K. Walker, P. Gilchrist et al. 2001. "Outcome in Patients with Eating Disorders: A 5–Year Study." *Lancet* 357: 1254–57.

Berkman, L., and I. Kawachi. 2000. *Social Epidemiology.* New York: Oxford University Press.

Bevier, P. J., M. A. Chiasson, R. T. Heffernan et al. 1995. "Women at a Sexually Transmitted Disease Clinic Who Reported Same-Sex Contact: Their HIV Seroprevalence and Risk Behaviors." *American Journal of Public Health* 85: 1366–71.

Black, D. R., editor. 1991. *Eating Disorders among Athletes.* Reston, Va.: American Alliance for Health, Physical Education, Recreation and Dance.

Bloor, M. 1995. *The Sociology of HIV Transmission.* Newbury Park, Calif.: Sage.

Bogdan, R. and S. J. Taylor. 1989. "Relationships with Severely Disabled People: The Social Construction of Humanness." *Social Problems* 36: 135–48.

Bond, L. S. 1992. "Street Children and AIDS: Is Postponement of Sexual Involvement a Realistic Alternative to the Prevention of Sexually Transmitted Diseases?" *Environment and Urbanization* 4: 150–57.

Borchert, J., and C. A. Rickabaugh. 1995. "When Illness is Perceived as Controllable: The Effects of Gender and Mode of Transmission on AIDS-Related Stigma." *Sex Roles* 33: 657–68.

Bordo, S. R. 1993. *Unbearable Weight: Feminism, Western Culture, and the Body.* Berkeley: University of California Press.

———. 1999. *The Male Body: A New Look at Men in Public and Private.* New York: Farrar Straus Giroux.

Borman, A. M., S. Paulous, and F. Clavel. 1996. "Resistance of Human-Immunodeficiency-Virus Type 1 to Protease Inhibitors: Selection of Resistance Mutations in the Presence and Absence of the Drug." *Journal of General Virology* 77(Part 3): 419–26.

Bourdieu, P. 1990. *The Logic of Practice.* Stanford, Calif.: Stanford University Press.

Boyd, R. L. 1989. "Racial Differences in Childlessness: A Centennial Review." *Sociological Perspectives* 2: 183–99.

Brady M. 1999. "Female Genital Mutilation: Complications and Risk of HIV Transmission." *AIDS Patient Care and Sexually Transmitted Diseases* 13: 709–16.

Breitbart, V., W. Chavkin, and P. Wise. 1994. "The Accessibility of Drug Treatment for Pregnant Women: A Survey of Programs in Five Cities." *American Journal of Public Health.* 84: 1658–61.

Brogan, D., E. Frank, L. Elon et al. 1999. "Harassment of Lesbians as Medical Students and Physicians." *JAMA* 282: 1290–92.

Brown, L. J., and V. Lazar. 1998. "Differences in Net Incomes of Male and Female Owner General Practitioners." *Journal of the American Dental Association* 129: 373–78.

Brown, P. 1995. "Naming and Framing: The Social Construction of Diagnosis and Illness." *Journal of Health and Social Behavior* (Extra Issue): 34–52.

Browne, J., and V. Minichiello. 1996. "Condoms: Dilemmas of Caring and Autonomy in Heterosexual Safe Sex Practices." *Venereology: Interdisciplinary International Journal of Sexual Health* 9: 24–33.

Brownworth, V., and S. Raffo. 1999. *Restricted Access: Lesbians on Disability.* Seattle, Wash.: Seal Press.

Brozan, N. 1978. "Training Linked to Disruption of Female Reproductive Cycle." *NYT*, April 17.

Brumberg, J. J. 1997. *The Body Project: An Intimate History of American Girls.* New York: Vintage Books.

Buckley, T., and A. Gottlieb. 1988. "A Critical Appraisal of Theories of Menstrual Symbolism." Pp. 3–50 in *Blood Magic: The Anthropology of Menstruation*, edited by T. Buckley and A. Gottlieb. Berkeley: University of California Press.

Bullard, D. G., and S. E. Knight. 1981. *Sexuality and Physical Disability: Personal Perspectives.* St. Louis: Mosby.

Bullough, V., and M. Voght. 1973. "Women, Menstruation and Nineteenth-Century Medicine." *Bulletin of the History of Medicine* 47: 66–82.

Burckes-Miller, M. E., and D. R. Black. 1991. "College Athletes and Eating Disorders: A Theoretical Context." Pp. 11–26 in *Eating Disorders among Athletes*, edited by D. R. Black. Reston, Va.: American Alliance for Health, Physical Education, Recreation and Dance.

Bush, T. L. 1992. "Feminine Forever Revisited: Menopausal Hormone Therapy in the 1990s." *JWH* 1: 1–4.

Butler, J. 1993. *Bodies that Matter: On the Discursive Limits of "Sex."* New York and London: Routledge.

Calderone, K. L. 1990. "The Influence of Gender on the Frequency of Pain and Sedative Medication Administered to Postoperative Patients." *Sex Roles* 23: 713–25.

Caldwell, J. C., and P. Caldwell. 1996. "The African AIDS Epidemic." *Scientific American* 274(3): 62–63, 66–68.

Callahan, J. C., editor. 1993. *Menopause: A Midlife Passage.* Bloomington: Indiana University Press.

Campbell, C. A. 1991. "Prostitution, AIDS and Preventive Health Behavior." *Social Science and Medicine* 32: 1367–78.

———. 1995. "Male Gender Roles and Sexuality: Implications for Women's AIDS Risk and Prevention." *Social Science and Medicine* 41: 197–210.

Candib, L. M. 1988. "Ways of Knowing in Family Medicine: Contributions from a Feminist Perspective." *Family Medicine* 20: 133–36.

———. 1995. *Medicine and the Family: A Feminist Perspective.* New York: Basic Books.

Cauley, J. A., D. M. Black, E. Barrett Connor et al. 2001. "Effect of Hormone Replacement Therapy on Clinical Fractures and Height Loss: The Heart and Estrogen/Progestin Replacement Study (HERS)." *American Journal of Medicine* 110: 442–50.

Cauvin, H. E. 2001. "How Rush to Manhood Scars Young Africans." *NYT*, August 6.

Charmaz, K. 1991. *Good Days, Bad Days: The Self in Chronic Illness and Time.* New Brunswick, N.J.: Rutgers University Press.

———. 1995. "Identity Dilemmas of Chronically Ill Men." Pp. 266–91 in *Men's Health and Illness: Gender, Power and the Body,* edited by D. Sabo and D. F. Gordon. Newbury Park, Calif.: Sage.

Chase, C. 1998. "Hermaphrodites with Attitude: Mapping the Emergence of Intersex Political Activism." *GLQ: A Journal of Gay and Lesbian Studies* 4: 189–211.

———. 2000. "Genital Surgery on Children below the Age of Consent: Intersex Genital Mutilation." Pp. 452–58 in *Psychological Perspectives on Human Sexuality,* edited by L. Szuchman and F. Muscarella. New York: John Wiley and Sons.

Chatterjee, N., and N. E. Riley. 2001. "Planning an Indian Modernity: The Gendered Politics of Fertility Control." *Signs* 26: 811–45.

Chavkin, W., editor. 1994. *Double Exposure: Women's Health Hazards on the Job and at Home.* New York: Monthly Review Press.

Chesney, M. 2000. "Factors Affecting Adherence to Antiretroviral Therapy." *Clinical Infectious Diseases* 30(Suppl. 2): S171–76.

Chrisler, J. C., and K. B. Levy. 1990. "The Media Construct a Menstrual Monster: A Content Analysis of PMS Articles in the Popular Press." *Women and Health* 16: 69–71.

Christakis, D. A., E. Harvey, and D. M Zerr et al. 2000. "A Trade-Off Analysis of Routine Newborn Circumcision." *Journal of the Ambulatory Pediatric Association* (Supplement) 105: 246–49.

Chu, S. Y., and P. M. Wortley. 1995. "Epidemiology of HIV/AIDS in Women." Pp. 1–12 in *HIV Infection in Women,* edited by H. Minkoff, J. A. DeHovitz, and A. Duerr. New York: Raven Press.

Clare, E. 1999. "Flirting with You: Some Notes on Isolation and Connection." Pp. 127–135 in *Restricted Access: Lesbians on Disability,* edited by V. Brownworth and S. Raffo. Seattle, Wash.: Seal Press.

Clarke, A. E., and V. L. Olesen, editors. 1999a. *Revisioning Women, Health, and Healing: Feminist, Cultural, and Technoscience Perspectives.* New York: Routledge.

———. 1999b. "Revising, Diffracting, Acting." Pp. 3–48 in *Revisioning Women, Health, and Healing: Feminist, Cultural, and Technoscience Perspectives,* edited by A. E. Clarke and V. L. Olesen. New York: Routledge.

Coale, A. J., and J. Banister. 1994. "Five Decades of Missing Females in China." *Demography* 31: 459–79.

Cohen, S. M., E. O. Mitchell, V. Oleson et al. 1994. "From Female Disease to Women's Health: New Educational Paradigms." Pp. 50–55 in *Reframing Women's Health,* by A. J. Dan. Newbury Park, Calif.: Sage.

Collins, C. 2000. "Can an HIV Vaccine Help in HIV Prevention?" Center for AIDS Prevention Studies, University of California San Francisco Web site.

Collins, P. Hill. 1990. *Black Feminist Thought: Knowledge, Consciousness, and the Politics of Empowerment.* Boston: Unwin Hyman.

Connell, R. W. 1995. *Masculinities.* Berkeley: University of California Press.

Connell, R. W., M. D. Davis, and G. W. Dowsett. 1993. "A Bastard of a Life: Homosexual Desire and Practice among Men in Working-Class Milieux." *Australia and New Zealand Journal of Sociology* 29: 112–35.

Connell, R. W., and Susan Kippax. 1990. "Sexuality in the AIDS Crisis: Patterns of Sexual Practice and Pleasure in a Sample of Australian Gay and Bisexual Men." *Journal of Sex Research* 27: 167–98.

Cooley, E., and T. Toray. 2001. "Body Image and Personality Predictors of Eating Disorder Symptoms during the College Years." *International Journal of Eating Disorders* 30: 28–36.

Cooper, E. B. 1995. "Historical and Analytical Overview of Policy Issues Affecting Women Living with AIDS: A Blueprint for Learning from Our Past." *Bulletin of the New York Academy of Medicine* 72(Summer Supp. 1): 283–99.

Cooper, S., and E. Glazer. 1998. *Choosing Assisted Reproduction: Social, Emotional, and Ethical Considerations.* Indianapolis: Perspectives Press.

Cooper-Patrick, L., J. J. Gallo, J. J. Gonzalez et al. 1999. "Race, Gender, and Partnership in the Physician-Patient Relationship." *JAMA* 282: 583–89.

Corbin, J. M., and A. Strauss. 1988. *Unending Work and Care: Managing Chronic Illness at Home.* San Francisco: Jossey-Bass.

Corea, G. 1992. *The Invisible Epidemic: The Story of Women and AIDS.* New York: HarperPerennial.

Coulter, I., P. Jacobson, and L. E. Parker. 2000. "Sharing the Mantle of Primary Female Care: Physicians, Nurse Practitioners, and Physician Assistants." *JAMWA* 55: 100–3.

Crossette, B. 2001. "Cheaper AIDS Drugs Pose More Dangers in Africa." *NYT,* April 1.

Crystal, S., and M. Jackson. 1992. "Health Care and the Social Construction of AIDS: The Impact of Disease Definitions." Pp. 163–80 in J. Huber and B. E. Schneider, eds., *The Social Context of AIDS.* Newbury Park, Calif.: Sage.

Dan, A. J. 1994. *Reframing Women's Health.* Newbury Park, Calif.: Sage.

D'aoust, V. 1999. "Complications: The Deaf Community, Disability and Being a Lesbian Mom: A Conversation with Myself." Pp. 115–126 in *Restricted Access: Lesbians on Disability,* edited by V. Brownworth and S. Raffo. Seattle, Wash.: Seal Press.

Daum, Meghan. 1996. "Safe-Sex Lies." *NYT Magazine,* January 21.

Davis, F. 1972. *Illness, Interaction and the Self.* Belmont, Calif.: Wadsworth.

Davis, K. 1995. *Reshaping the Female Body: The Dilemma of Cosmetic Surgery.* New York: Routledge.

——. 1988. *Power under the Microscope.* Dordrecht, the Netherlands: Foris.

Dean, M., M. Carrington, C. Winkler et al. 1996. "Genetic Restriction of HIV-1 Infection and Progression to AIDS by a Deletion Allele of the *CKR5* Structural Gene." *Science* 273(Sept. 27): 1856–62.

Deegan, M. J. 1985. "Multiple Minority Groups: A Case Study of Physically Disabled Women." Pp. 37–55 in *Women and Disability: The Double Handicap,* edited by M. J. Deegan and N. A. Brooks. New Brunswick, N.J.: Transaction Books.

Deegan, M. J., and N. A. Brooks, editors. 1985. *Women and Disability: The Double Handicap.* New Brunswick, N.J.: Transaction Books.

DeHaan, C. B., and J. L. Wallander. 1988. "Self-Concept, Sexual Knowledge and Attitudes, and Parental Support in the Sexual Adjustment of Women with Early- and Late-Onset Physical Disability." *Archives of Sexual Behavior* 17: 145–61.

Delany, S. R. 1991. "Straight Talk/Street Talk." *Differences* 3(Summer): 21–38.

Diamond, T. 1992. *Making Gray Gold: Narratives from Inside Nursing Homes.* Chicago: University of Chicago Press.

Dickson, G. L. 1990. "A Feminist Poststructuralist Analysis of the Knowledge of Menopause." *Advances in Nursing Science* 12: 15–31.

Dixon-Mueller, R. 1994. "Abortion Policy and Women's Health in Developing Countries." Pp. 191–210 in E. Fee and N. Krieger, eds., *Women's Health, Politics, and Power*. Amityville, N.Y.: Baywood.

Dorrington, R., D. Bourne, and D. Bradshaw et al. 2001. "The Impact of HIV/AIDS on Adult Mortality in South Africa." Medical Research Council Web site.

Douglas, M. 1966. *Purity and Danger: An Analysis of the Concepts of Pollution and Taboo*. London: Routledge & Kegan Paul.

Doyal, L. 2001. "Sex, Gender, and Health: The Need for a New Approach." *BMJ* 323: 1061–63.

Drachman, V. 1984. *Hospital with a Heart*. Ithaca, N.Y.: Cornell University Press.

Draper, E. 1993. "Fetal Exclusion Policies and Gendered Constructions of Suitable Work." *Social Problems* 40: 90–107.

Dreger, A. Domurat. 1998. *Hermaphrodites and the Medical Invention of Sex*. Cambridge, Mass.: Harvard University Press.

Duerr, A., and G. E. Howe. 1995. "Contraception." Pp. 157–72 in *HIV Infection in Women*, edited by H. Minkoff, J. A. DeHovitz, and A. Duerr. New York: Raven Press.

Dugger, C. W. 1996. "Genital Ritual is Unyielding in Africa." *NYT*, October 5.

Dworkin, S., and M. A. Messner. 1999. "Just Do . . . What? Sport, Bodies, Gender." Pp. 341–61 in *Revisioning Gender*, edited by M. M. Ferree, J. Lorber, and B. B. Hess. Thousand Oaks, Calif.: Sage.

Ehrenreich, B., and D. English. 1973. *Complaints and Disorders: The Sexual Politics of Sickness*. N.Y.: Feminist Press.

Ekstrand, M. L., R. D. Stall, J. P. Paul et al. 1999. "Gay Men Report High Rates of Unprotected Anal Sex with Partners of Unknown or Discordant HIV Status." *AIDS* 13: 1525–33.

El Dareer, A. 1982. *Woman, Why Do You Weep? Circumcision and its Consequences*. London: Zed Books.

Elias, C., and Coggins, C. 2001. "Acceptability Research on Female-Controlled Barrier Methods to Prevent Heterosexual Transmission of HIV: Where Have We Been? Where Are We Going?" *JWH* 10: 163–73.

Ericksen, K. Paige. 1995. "Female Circumcision among Egyptian Women." *Women's Health: Research on Gender, Behavior, and Policy* 1: 309–28.

Espinoza, P., I. Bouchard, and P. Ballian. 1988. "Has the Open Sale of Syringes Modified the Syringe-Exchanging Habits of Drug Addicts?" Abstract 8522 in *Final Program and Abstracts of the IV International Conference on AIDS*. Stockholm.

Ettorre, E., and E. Riska. 1995. *Gendered Moods: Psychotropics and Society*. New York: Routledge.

Fausto-Sterling, Anne.1985. *Myths of Gender: Biological Theories about Women and Men*. New York: Basic Books.

———. 2000. *Sexing the Body: Gender Politics and the Construction of Sexuality*. New York: Basic Books.

Featherstone, M., M. Hepworth, and B. S. Turner, editors. 1991. *The Body: Social Process and Cultural Theory*. Newbury Park, Calif.: Sage.

Fee, E. and N. Krieger (eds.). 1994. *Women's Health, Politics, and Power*. Amityville, N.Y.: Baywood.

Fennema, K., D. L. Meyer, and N. Owen. 1990. "Sex of Physician: Patients' Preferences and Stereotypes." *Journal of Family Practice* 30: 441–46.

Figert, A. E. 1995. "The Three Faces of PMS: The Professional, Gendered and Scientific Structuring of a Psychiatric Disorder." *Social Problems* 42: 56–73.

Fine, M., and A. Asch. 1985. "Disabled Women: Sexism without the Pedestal." Pp. 6–22 in *Women and Disability: The Double Handicap,* edited by M. J. Deegan and N. A. Brooks. New Brunswick, N.J.: Transaction Books.

Fine, M., and A. Asch, editors. 1988. *Women with Disabilities: Essays in Psychology, Culture, and Politics.* Philadelphia: Temple University Press.

Fisher, S. 1986. *In the Patient's Best Interest: Women and the Politics of Medical Decisions.* New Brunswick, N.J.: Rutgers University Press.

———. 1994. "Is Care a Remedy? The Case of Nurse Practitioners." Pp. 301–29 in *Reframing Women's Health,* by A. J. Dan. Newbury Park, Calif.: Sage.

———. 1995. *Nursing Wounds: Nurse Practitioners, Doctors, Women Patients, and the Negotiation of Meaning.* New Brunswick, N.J.: Rutgers University Press.

Flint, M. 1982. "Male and Female Menopause: A Cultural Put-on." Pp. 363–75 in *Changing Perspectives on Menopause,* edited by A. M. Voda, M. Dinnerstein, and S. R. O'Donnell. Austin: University of Texas Press.

Flint, M., and R. S. Samil. 1990. "Cultural and Subcultural Meaning of the Menopause." Pp. 134–48 in *Multidisciplinary Perspectives on Menopause,* edited by M. Flint, F. Kronenberg, and W. Utian. New York: New York Academy of Sciences.

Fontanet, A.L., J. Saba, J. Chandelying et al. 1998. "Protection Against Sexually Transmitted Diseases by Granting Sex Workers in Thailand the Choice of Using the Male or Female Condom: Results from a Randomized Controlled Trial." *AIDS* 12: 1851–59.

Foster, J. 1996. "Menstrual Time: The Sociocognitive Mapping of 'The Menstrual Cycle.'" *Sociological Forum* 11: 523–47.

Frackiewicz, E. J., and T. M. Shiovitz. 2001. "Evaluation and Management of Premenstrual Syndrome and Premenstrual Dysphoric Disorder." *Journal of American Pharmacy Association* 41: 437–47.

Frank, G. 1988. "On Embodiment: A Case Study of Congenital Limb Deficiency in American Culture." Pp. 41–71 in *Women with Disabilities: Essays in Psychology, Culture, and Politics,* edited by M. Fine and A. Asch. Philadelphia: Temple University Press.

Frank, R. 1931. "The Hormonal Causes of Premenstrual Tension." *Archives of Neurology and Psychiatry.* 26: 1053–57.

Franks, P., and C. M. Clancy. 1993. "Physician Gender Bias in Clinical Decision-Making: Screening for Cancer in Primary Care." *Medical Care* 31: 213–18.

Freidson, Eliot. 1970a. *Profession of Medicine.* New York: Dodd Mead.

———. 1970b. *Professional Dominance: The Social Structure of Medical Care.* New York: Atherton.

———. 1986. *Professional Powers.* Chicago: University of Chicago Press.

———. 1989. *Medical Work in America.* New Haven, Conn.: Yale University Press.

Fussell, S. 1993. "Body Builder Americanus." *Michigan Quarterly Review* 32: 577–96.

Gallagher, H. G. 1985. *FDR's Splendid Deception.* New York: Dodd Mead.

Gamble, V. 1982. "Vanessa Gamble: Tomorrow's Physicians, Tomorrow's Policy-Maker." Pp. 242–61 in *In Her Own Words: Oral Histories of Women Physicians,* edited by R. M. Morantz, C. S. Pomerlau, and C. H. Fenichel. Westport, Conn.: Greenwood Press.

Gannon, L., and B. Ekstrom. 1993. "Attitudes toward Menopause: The Influence of Sociocultural Paradigms." *Psychology of Women Quarterly* 17: 275–88.

Gartner, R. 1990. "The Victims of Homicide: A Temporal and Cross-National Comparison." *American Sociological Review* 55: 92–106.

Genuis, S. J., and S. K. Genuis. 1996. "Orgasm without Organisms: Science or Propaganda?" *Clinical Pediatrics* 35: 10–17.

Gerschick, T. J., and A. S. Miller. 1994. "Gender Identities at the Crossroads of Masculinity and Physical Disability." *Masculinities* 2: 34–55.

Gibbs, J. T., editor. 1988. *Young, Black and Male in America: An Endangered Species.* Dover, Mass.: Auburn House.

Gill, C. J. 1994. "When is a Woman Not a Woman." *Sexuality and Disability* 12: 117–20.

Gitlin, M. J., and R. O. Pasnau. 1989. "Psychiatric Syndromes Linked to Reproductive Function in Women: A Review of Current Knowledge." *American Journal of Psychiatry* 146: 1413–21.

Gladwell, M. 2000. "John Rock's Error." *New Yorker Magazine*, March 13, pp. 52–63.

Glass, J., and T. Fujimoto. 1994. "Housework, Paid Work, and Depression among Husbands and Wives." *Journal of Health and Social Behavior* 35: 179–91.

Glazer, N. 1990. "The Home as Workshop: Women as Amateur Nurses and Medical Care Providers." *Gender & Society* 4: 479–99.

———. 1991. "'Between a Rock and Hard Place': Women's Professional Organizations in Nursing and Class, Racial, and Ethnic Inequalities." *Gender & Society* 5: 351–72.

Goldberg, C. 1995. "Suicide's Husband is Indicted: Diary Records Pain of 2 Lives." *NYT*, December 15.

Goldman, R. 1998. *Questioning Circumcision: A Jewish Perspective.* New York: Vanguard.

Goldstein, D. 2000. "'When Ovaries Retire': Contrasting Women's Experiences with Feminist and Medical Models of Menopause." *Health* 4: 309–23.

Goldstein, N. 1995. "Lesbians and the Medical Profession: HIV/AIDS and the Pursuit of Visibility." *Women's Studies* 24: 531–52.

Goldstein, N., and J. L. Manlowe, editors. 1997. *The Gender Politics of HIV/AIDS in Women.* New York: New York University Press.

Gollaher, D. L. 2000. *Circumcision: A History of the World's Most Controversial Surgery.* New York: Basic Books.

Golub, S. 1992. *Periods: From Menarche to Menopause.* Newbury Park, Calif.: Sage.

Gómez, C. A. 1995. "Lesbians at Risk for HIV: The Unresolved Debate." Pp. 19–31 in *AIDS, Identity, and Community: The HIV Epidemic and Lesbians and Gay Men,* edited by G. M. Herek and B. Greene. Newbury Park, Calif.: Sage.

Goode, E. 2001. "With Fears Fading, More Gays Spurn Old Preventive Message." *NYT*, August 19.

Greenhalgh, Susan. 2001. "Fresh Winds in Beijing: Chinese Feminists Speak Out on the One-Child Policy and Women's Lives." *Signs* 26: 847–86.

Greenhalgh, S., and J. Li. 1995. "Engendering Reproductive Policy and Practice in Peasant China: For a Feminist Demography of Reproduction." *Signs* 20: 601–41.

Greer, G. 1991. *The Change: Women, Aging and the Menopause.* New York: Fawcett Columbine.

Gremillion, H. 2002. "In Fitness and in Health: Crafting Bodies in the Treatment of Anorexia Nervosa." *Signs* 27: 381–414.

Griffiths, F. 1999. "Women's Control and Choice Regarding HRT." *Social Science and Medicine* 49: 469–81.

Grinstead, O., B. Zack, and B. Faigeles et al. 1999. "Reducing Postrelease HIV Risk among Male Prison Inmates: A Peer-Led Intervention." *Criminal Justice and Behavior* 26: 453–65.

Grodstein, F., J. E. Manson, and M. J. Stampfer. 2001. "Postmenopausal Hormone Use and Secondary Prevention of Coronary Events in the Nurses' Health Study." *Annals of Internal Medicine* 135: 1–8.

Gruenbaum, E. 2000. *The Female Circumcision Controversy: An Anthropological Perspective*. Philadelphia: University of Pennsylvania Press.

Grumbach, K., and J. Coffman. 1998. "Physicians and Non-Physician Clinicians: Complements or Competitors?" *JAMA* 280: 825–26.

Guinan, M. E. 1988. "PMS or Perifollicular Phase Euphoria?" *JAMWA* 43: 91–92.

Gullette, M. Morganroth. 1993. "All Together Now: The New Sexual Politics of Midlife Bodies." *Michigan Quarterly Review* 32: 669–95.

Gutiérrez, L., H. J. Oh, and M. Rogers Gillmore. 2000. "Toward and Understand of (Em)Power(Ment) for HIV/AIDS Prevention with Adolescent Women." *Sex Roles* 42: 581–611.

Hall, J. A., A. M. Epstein, M. L. DeCiantis et al. 1993. "Physicians' Liking for Their Patients: More Evidence for the Role of Affect in Medical Care." *Health Psychology* 12: 140–46.

Hall, J. A., J. T. Irish, D. L. Roter et al. 1994. "Gender in Medical Encounters: An Analysis of Physician and Patient Communication in a Primary Care Setting." *Health Psychology* 13: 382–92.

Hall, J. A., and D. L. Roter. 1995. "Patient Gender and Communication with Physicians: Results of a Community-Based Study." *Women's Health: Research on Gender, Behavior, and Policy* 1: 77–95.

Halperin, D. T., and R. C. Bailey. 1999. "Male Circumcision and HIV Infection: 10 Years and Counting." *Lancet* 354: 1813–15.

Hammonds, E. 1992. "Missing Persons: African American Women, AIDS and the History of Disease." *Radical America* 24: 7–23.

Haraway, D. 1989. "The Biopolitics of Postmodern Bodies: Determinations of Self in Immune System Discourse." *Differences* 1(Winter): 1–43.

Harding, S. 1986. *The Science Question in Feminism*. Ithaca, N.Y.: Cornell University Press.

Harlow, S. D., K. Bainbridge, D. Howard et al. 1999. "Methods and Measures: Emerging Strategies in Women's Health Research." *JWH* 8: 139–44.

Harrison, M. 1983. *A Woman in Residence*. New York: Penguin.

———. 1985. *Self-Help for Premenstrual Syndrome*. New York: Random House.

———. 1990. "Women as Other: The Premise of Medicine." *JAMWA* 45: 225–26.

———. 1994. "Women's Health: New Models of Care and a New Academic Discipline." Pp. 79–90 in *Reframing Women's Health*, by A. J. Dan. Newbury Park, Calif.: Sage.

Hartgers, C., E. van Ameijden, E, J. van den Hoek et al. 1992. "Needle Sharing and Participation in the Amsterdam Syringe Exchange Among HIV-Seronegative Injecting Drug Users." *Public Health Reports.* 107: 675–81.

Haug, M., and B. Lavin. 1983. *Consumerism in Medicine: Challenging Physician Authority*. Newbury Park, Calif.: Sage.

Haynes, S. G., B. S. Lynch, R. Biegel et al. 2000. "Women's Health and the Environment: Innovations in Science and Policy." *JWH* 9: 245–73.

Healy, B. 1991. "The Yentl Syndrome." *New England Journal of Medicine* 325: 274–76.

Herdt, G. and S. Lindenbaum (eds.). 1992. *The Time of AIDS: Social Analysis, Theory, and Method*. Newbury Park, Calif.: Sage.

Herzog, D. B., K. L. Newman, C. J. Yeh, and M. Warshaw. 1992. "Body Image Satisfaction in Homosexual and Heterosexual Women." *International Journal of Eating Disorders* 11: 391–96.

Hill, S. A., and M. K. Zimmerman. 1995. "Valiant Girls and Vulnerable Boys: The Impact of Gender and Race on Mothers' Caregiving for Chronically Ill Children." *Journal of Marriage and the Family* 57: 43–53.

Hillyer, B. 1993. *Feminism and Disability*. Norman: University of Oklahoma Press.

Hine, D. Clark. 1985. "Co-laborers in the Work of the Lord: Nineteenth-Century Black Physicians." Pp.107–20 in *"Send Us a Lady Physician": Women Doctors in America, 1835–1920*, edited by R. J. Abram. New York: Norton.

———. 1989. *Black Women in White: Racial Conflict and Cooperation in the Nursing Profession, 1890–1950*. New York: Routledge.

Hockenberry, J. 1995. *Moving Violations: War Zones, Wheelchairs, and Declarations of Independence*. New York: Hyperion.

Hoffmann, J. C. 1982. "Biorhythms in Human Reproduction: The Not-So-Steady States." *Signs* 7: 829–44.

Hoffman, L. A. 1995. *Covenant of Blood: Circumcision and Gender in Rabbinic Judaism*. Chicago: University of Chicago Press.

Hogben, M., and J. S. St. Lawrence. 2000. "HIV/STD Risk Reduction Interventions in Prison Settings." *JWH* 9: 587–92.

Hollibaugh, A. 1995. "Lesbian Denial and Lesbian Leadership in the AIDS Epidemic: Bravery and Fear in the Construction of Lesbian Geography of Risk." Pp. 219–30 in *Women Resisting AIDS: Feminist Strategies of Empowerment*, edited by B. E. Schneider and N. E. Stoller. Philadelphia: Temple University Press.

Hubbard, R. 1990. *The Politics of Women's Biology*. New Brunswick, N.J.: Rutgers University Press.

Huber, J. and B. E. Schneider, editors. 1992. *The Social Context of AIDS*. Newbury Park, Calif.: Sage.

Hughes, E. C. 1971. "Dilemmas and Contradictions of Status." Pp. 141–50 in *The Sociological Eye*. Chicago: Aldine Atherton.

Hunter, D. J., B. N. Maggwa, J. K. Mati et al. 1994. "Sexual Behavior, Sexually Transmitted Diseases, Male Circumcision and Risk of HIV Infection among Women in Nairobi, Kenya." *AIDS* 8: 93–99.

Hutchinson, M., and M. Shannon. 1993. "Reproductive Health and Counseling." Pp. 47–65 in A. Kurth, ed., *Until the Cure: Caring for Women with HIV*. New Haven, Conn.: Yale University Press.

Idler, E. L., and S. V. Kasl. 1992. "Religion, Disability, Depression, and the Timing of Death." *American Journal of Sociology* 97: 1052–79.

IOM (Institute of Medicine). 2001. *Health and Behavior: The Interplay of Biological, Behavioral, and Societal Influences*. Washington, D.C.: National Academy Press.

James, M. S. 2001. "Till Sickness Do We Part Study: Husbands More Likely to Divorce Ill Spouses." ABC News Online May 12.

James, S. A. 1994. "Reconciling Human Rights and Cultural Relativism: The Case of Female Circumcision." *Bioethics* 8 (Nov. 1): 1–26.

———. 1998. "Shades of Othering: Reflections on Female Circumcision/Genital Mutilation." *Signs* 23: 1031–48.

Jason, J., B. L. Evatt, and Hemophilia-AIDS Collaborative Study Group. 1990. "Pregnancies in Human Immunodeficiency Virus-Infected Sex Partners of Hemophilic Men." *American Journal of Diseases of Children* 144: 485–90.

Jenkins, S. R. 2000. "Introduction to the Special Issue: Defining Gender, Relationships, and Power." *Sex Roles* 42: 751–80.

Johnson, K., and E. Hoffman. 1994. "Women's Health and Curriculum Transformation: The Role of Medical Specialization." Pp. 27–39 in *Reframing Women's Health*, by A. J. Dan. Newbury Park, Calif.: Sage.

Jones, E., and J. Darroch Forrest. 1985. "Teenage Pregnancy in Developed Countries: Determinants and Policy Implications." *Family Planning Perspectives* 17: 53–63.

Kahn J. O., J. N. Martin, M. E. Roland et al. 2001. "Feasibility of Postexposure Prophylaxis (PEP) against Human Immunodeficiency Virus Infection after Sexual or Injection Drug Use Exposure: San Francisco PEP Study." *Journal of Infectious Diseases* 183: 707–14.

Kane, S., and T. Mason. 1992. "'IV Drug Users' and 'Sex Partners': The Limits of Epidemiological Categories and the Ethnography of Risk." Pp. 199–222 in G. Herdt and S. Lindenbaum, eds., *The Time of AIDS: Social Analysis, Theory, and Method*. Newbury Park, Calif.: Sage.

Kantor, E. 1998. "HIV Transmission and Prevention in Prisons." Center for AIDS Prevention Studies, University of California San Francisco Web site.

Kasper, A. S. 1995. "The Social Construction of Breast Loss and Reconstruction." *Women's Health Research on Gender, Behavior, and Policy*. 3: 197–219.

Kaw, E. 1998. "Medicalization of Racial Features: Asian-American Women and Cosmetic Surgery." Pp. 147–83 in *The Politics of Women's Bodies: Sexuality, Appearance and Behavior*, edited by R. Weitz. New York: Oxford University Press.

Kaye, L. W., and J. S. Applegate. 1990. *Men as Caregivers to the Elderly: Understanding and Aiding Unrecognized Family Support*. Lexington, Mass.: Lexington Books.

Kegeles, S. M., R. B. Hays, L. M. Pollack et al. 1999. "Mobilizing Young Gay Men for HIV Prevention: A Two-Community Study." *AIDS* 13: 1753–62.

Kelly, J. A. 1995a. "Advances in HIV/AIDS Education and Prevention." *Family Relations* 44: 345–52.

———. 1995b. *Changing HIV Risk Behavior: Practical Strategies*. New York: Guilford.

Kelly, J. A, J. S. St. Lawrence, Y. E. Diaz et al. 1991. "HIV Risk Behavior Reduction Following Intervention with Key Opinion Leaders of a Population: An Experimental Community-Level Analysis." *American Journal of Public Health* 81: 168–71.

Kelly, M. 1996. "Accentuate the Negative." *The New Yorker*, April 1, 44–48.

Kemper, T. D. 1990. *Social Structure and Testosterone: Explorations of the Sociobiosocial Chain*. New Brunswick, N.J.: Rutgers University Press.

Kennamer, J. D., J. Honnold, J. Bradford et al. 2000. "Differences in Disclosure of Sexuality among African American and White Gay/Bisexual Men: Implications for HIV/AIDS Prevention." *AIDS Education and Prevention* 12: 519–31.

Kennedy, M. B., M. I. Scarlett, A. C. Duerr et al. 1995. "Assessing HIV Risk among Women Who Have Sex with Women: Scientific and Communication Issues." *JAMWA* 50: 103–7.

Kessler, S. J. 1998. *Lessons from the Intersexed*. New Brunswick, N.J.: Rutgers University Press.

Kessler, S. J., and W. McKenna. 1985. *Gender: An Ethnomethodological Approach*. Chicago: University of Chicago Press.

Killoran, C. 1994. "Women with Disabilities Having Children: It's Our Right, Too." *Sexuality and Disability* 12: 121–26.

Kimmel, M. 2001. "The Kindest Uncut: Feminism, Judaism and My Son's Foreskin." *Tikkun* (May–June): 43–48.

Kimmel, M., and M. P. Levine. 1991. "A Hidden Factor in AIDS: 'Real' Men's Hypersexuality." *Los Angeles Times*, June 3.

King, D. 1990. "Prostitutes as Pariah in the Age of AIDS: A Content Analysis of Coverage of Women Prostitutes in *The New York Times* and *The Washington Post* September 1985–April 1988." *Women and Health* 16: 135–76.

Kipnis, K., and M. Diamond. 1998. "Pediatric Ethics and the Surgical Assignment of Sex." *Journal of Clinical Ethics* 9: 398–410.

Kliewer, E. V., and K. R. Smith. 1995. "Breast Cancer Mortality among Immigrants in Australia and Canada." *Journal of the National Cancer Institute* 87: 1154–61.

Knight, C. 1991. *Blood Relations: Menstruation and the Origins of Culture*. New Haven, Conn.: Yale University Press.

Koch, L. 1990. "IVF—An Irrational Choice?" *Issues in Reproductive and Genetic Engineering* 3: 235–42.

Kocher, M. 1994. "Mothers with Disabilities." *Sexuality and Disability* 12: 127–34.

Koeske, R. Daimon. 1983. "Lifting the Curse of Menstruation: Toward a Feminist Perspective on the Menstrual Cycle." *Women and Health* 8(2–3): 1–15.

Kolata, G. 1991. "Hit Hard by AIDS Virus, Hemophiliacs Angrily Speak Out." *NYT*, December 25.

Kolb, C. 1985. "Assertive Training for Women with Visual Impairments." Pp. 87–94 in *Women and Disability: The Double Handicap*, edited by M. J. Deegan and N. A. Brooks. New Brunswick, N.J.: Transaction Books.

Koos, E. L. 1954. *The Health of Regionville*. New York: Columbia University Press.

Korvick, J. A., P. Stratton, C. Spino et al. 1996. "Women's Participation in AIDS Clinical Trials Group (ACTG) Trials in the USA: Enough or Still Too Few?" *JWH* 5: 129–36.

Kranczer, S. 1995. "U.S. Longevity Unchanged." *Statistical Bulletin* 76(3): 12–20.

Krieger, N. 1996. "Inequality, Diversity, and Health: Thoughts on 'Race/Ethnicity' and 'Gender.'" *JAMWA* 51: 133–36.

Kreiss J. K., and S. G. Hopkins. 1993. "The Association between Circumcision Status and Human Immunodeficiency Virus Infection among Homosexual Men." *Journal of Infectious Diseases* 168: 1404–8.

Kreuter, M. W., V. J. Strecher, R. Harris et al. 1995. "Are Patients of Women Physicians Screened More Aggressively? A Prospective Study of Physician Gender and Screening." *Journal of General Internal Medicine* 10: 119–25.

Kurth, A., editor. 1993. *Until the Cure: Caring for Women with HIV*. New Haven, Conn.: Yale University Press.

Lakoff, R. Tolmach. 1989. "Review Essay: Woman and Disability." *Feminist Studies* 15: 365–75.

Laumann, E. O., C. M. Masi, and E. W. Zuckerman 1997. "Circumcision in the United States." *JAMA* 277: 1052–57.

Lawlor, D. A., S. Ebrahim, and G. Davey Smith. 2001. "Sex Matters: Secular and Geographical Trends in Sex Differences in Coronary Heart Disease Mortality." *BMJ* 323: 541–45.

Laws, S. 1983. "The Sexual Politics of Premenstrual Tension." *Women's Studies International Forum* 6: 19–31.

———. 1990. *Issues of Blood: The Politics of Menstruation.* London: Macmillan.

Laws, S., V. Hey, and A. Egan. 1985. *Seeing Red: The Politics of Premenstrual Tension.* London: Hutchinson.

Lear, D. 1995. "Sexual Communication in the Age of AIDS: The Construction of Risk and Trust among Young Adults." *Social Science and Medicine* 41: 1311–23.

Lee. L. M., and P. L. Fleming. 2001. "Trends in Human Immunodeficiency Virus Diagnoses among Women in the United States, 1994–1998." *Journal of the American Medical Women's Association* 56: 94–99.

Lennane, K. J., and R. J. Lennane. 1973. "Alleged Psychogenic Disorders in Women—A Possible Manifestation of Sexual Prejudice." *New England Journal of Medicine* 288: 288–92.

Leonard, L. 2000a. "Interpreting Female Genital Cutting: Moving Beyond the Impasse." *Annual Review of Sex Research* 11: 158–91.

———. 2000b. " 'We Did It for Pleasure Only': Hearing Alternative Tales of Female Circumcision." *Qualitative Inquiry* 6: 212–28.

Levenson, J. D. 2000. "The New Enemies of Circumcision." *Commentary* 109 (March): 29–36.

Levesque-Lopman, L. 1988. *Claiming Reality: Phenomenology and Women's Experience.* Lanham, M.D.: Rowman & Littlefield.

Levine, M. P. 1992. "The Implications of Constructionist Theory for Social Research on the AIDS Epidemic among Gay Men." Pp. 185–98 in G. Herdt and S. Lindenbaum, eds., *The Time of AIDS: Social Analysis, Theory, and Method.* Newbury Park, Calif.: Sage.

Levine, M. P., and K. Siegel. 1992. "Unprotected Sex: Understanding Gay Men's Participation." Pp. 47–71 in in J. Huber and B. E. Schneider, eds., *The Social Context of AIDS.* Newbury Park, Calif.: Sage.

Lewis, D. K. 1995. "African-American Women at Risk: Notes on the Sociocultural Context of HIV Infection." Pp. 57–73 in *Women Resisting AIDS: Feminist Strategies of Empowerment*, edited by B. E. Schneider and N. E. Stoller. Philadelphia: Temple University Press.

Lewis, J. 1993. "Feminism, the Menopause and Hormone Replacement Therapy." *Feminist Review* 43: 38–56.

Lightfoot-Klein, H. 1989. *Prisoners of Ritual: An Odyssey into Female Circumcision in Africa.* New York: Harrington Park.

Lillard, L. A., and L. J. Waite. 1995. "'Til Death Do Us Part: Marital Disruption and Mortality." *American Journal of Sociology* 100: 1131–56.

Link, B. G., and J. Phelan. 1995. "Social Conditions as Fundamental Causes of Disease." *Journal of Health and Social Behavior* (Extra Issue): 80–94.

Litsky, F. 2001. "Diana Golden Brosnihan, Skier, Dies at 38." *NYT*, August 28.

Liu, R., W. A. Paxton, S. Choe et al. 1996. "Homozygous Defect in HIV–1 Coreceptor Accounts for Resistance of Some Multiply-Exposed Individuals to HIV–1 Infection." *Cell* 86: 367–77.

Lock, M. 1993. *Encounters with Aging: Mythologies of Menopause in Japan and North America*. Berkeley: University of California Press.

Lock, M., and P. Kaufert. 2001. "Menopause, Local Biologies and Cultures of Aging." *American Journal of Human Biology*. 13: 494–504.

Logue, B. J. 1991. "Taking Charge: Death Control as an Emergent Women's Issue." *Women's Health* 17: 97–121.

London, A., and A. Robles. 2000. "The Co-occurrence of Correct and Incorrect HIV Transmission Knowledge and Perceived Risk for HIV among Women of Childbearing Age in El Salvador." *Social Science and Medicine* 51: 1267–78.

Longino, C. F., Jr. 1988. "A Population Profile of Very Old Men and Women in the United States." *Sociological Quarterly* 29: 559–64.

Longman, J. 2001. "Knee Injuries Take a Toll on Many Female Athletes." *NYT*, March 29.

Lonsdale, S. 1990. *Women and Disability*. New York: St. Martin's Press.

Lorber, J. 1984. *Women Physicians: Careers, Status, and Power*. New York: Tavistock.

———. 1985. "More Women Physicians: Will It Mean More Humane Health Care?" *Social Policy* 16 (Summer): 50–54.

———. 1989. "Choice, Gift, or Patriarchal Bargain? Women's Consent to *In Vitro* Fertilization in Male Infertility." *Hypatia* 4: 23–36.

———. 1993b. "Why Women Physicians Will Never Be True Equals in the American Medical Profession." Pp. 62–97 in *Gender, Work and Medicine: Women and the Medical Division of Labor*, edited by E. Riska and K. Wegar. Newbury Park, Calif.: Sage.

Lorber, J., and L. Bandlamudi. 1993. "Dynamics of Marital Bargaining in Male Infertility." *Gender & Society* 7: 32–49.

Lorde, A. 1980. *The Cancer Journals*. San Francisco, Calif.: Aunt Lute Books.

Luciano, L. 2001. *Looking Good: Male Body Image in Modern America*. New York: Hill and Wang.

Lupton, D. 1993. "Risk as Moral Danger: The Social and Political Functions of Risk Discourse in Public Health." *International Journal of Health Services* 23: 425–35.

Lupton, D., S. McCarthy, and S. Chapman. 1995. "'Panic Bodies': Discourses on Risk and HIV Antibody Testing." *Sociology of Health and Illness* 17: 89–108.

Lurie, N., J. Slater, P. McGovern et al. 1993. "Preventive Care for Women: Does the Sex of the Physician Matter?" *New England Journal of Medicine* 329: 478–82.

MacPhail, C., and C. Campbell. 2001. "'I Think Condoms Are Good but, Aai, I Hate Those Things': Condom Use among Adolescents and Young People in a Southern African Township." *Social Science and Medicine* 52: 1613–27.

Mairs, N. 1986. *Plaintext*. Tucson: University of Arizona Press.

Mansfield, A., and B. McGinn. 1993. "Pumping Irony: The Muscular and the Feminine." Pp. 49–68 in *Body Matters: Essays on the Sociology of the Body*, edited by S. Scott and D. Morgan. London: Falmer Press.

Markens, S. 1996. "The Problematic of 'Experience': A Political and Cultural Critique of PMS." *Gender & Society* 10: 42–58.

Marks, N. F. 1988. "Does It Hurt to Care? Caregiving, Work-Family Conflict, and Midlife Well-Being." *Journal of Marriage and the Family* 60: 951–96.

Marseille, E., J. G. Kahn, K. Billinghurst and J. Saba. 2001. "Cost-Effectiveness of Female Condom in Preventing HIV and STDs in Commercial Sex Workers in Rural South Africa." *Social Science and Medicine*. 52: 135–48.

Marsiglio, W. 1988. "Commitment to Social Fatherhood: Predicting Adolescent Males' Intentions to Live with Their Child and Partner." *Journal of Marriage and the Family* 50: 427–41.

Martin, E. 1992. *The Woman in the Body: A Cultural Analysis of Reproduction.* Boston: Beacon Press.

Martin, S. C., R. M. Arnold, and R. M. Parker. 1988. "Gender and Medical Socialization." *Journal of Health and Social Behavior* 29: 333–43.

Masur, H., M. A. Michelis, G. P. Wormser et al. 1982. "Opportunistic Infection in Previously Healthy Women: Initial Manifestation of a Community-Acquired Cellular Immunodeficiency." *Annals of Internal Medicine* 97: 533–38.

Mbizvo, M. T., and M. T. Basset. 1996. "Reproductive Health and AIDS Prevention in Sub-Saharan Africa: The Case for Increased Male Participation." *Health Policy and Planning* 11: 84–92.

McClintock, M. K. 1971. "Menstrual Synchrony and Suppression." *Nature* 229: 244–45.

McCrea, F. B. 1986. "The Politics of Menopause: The 'Discovery' of a Deficiency Disease." Pp. 296–307 in *The Sociology of Health and Illness*, edited by P. Conrad and R. Kern. New York: St. Martin's Press.

McGovern, T., M. Davis, and M. B. Caschetta. 1994. "Inclusion of Women in AIDS Clinical Research: A Political and Legal Analysis." *JAMWA* 49: 102–04, 109.

McKee, M., and V. Shkolnikov. 2001. "Understanding the Toll of Premature Death among Men in Eastern Europe." *BMJ* 323: 1051–55.

McMillan, D. 1996. "Everything You Always Wanted to Know about Oral Sex." *San Francisco Bay Times*, January 25.

Melnick, S. L., R. Sherer, T. A. Louis et al. 1994. "Survival and Disease Progression According to Gender of Patients with HIV Infection." *JAMA* 272: 1915–21.

Melosh, B. 1982. *"The Physician's Hand": Work Culture and Conflict in American Nursing.* Philadelphia: Temple University Press.

Merrick, J. C., and R. H. Blank. 1993. *The Politics of Pregnancy: Policy Dilemmas in the Maternal–Fetal Relationship.* New York: Haworth.

Messing, K. 1997. "Women's Occupational Health: A Critical Review and Discussion of Current Issues." *Women's Health* 25: 39–68.

Messner, M. 1992. *Power at Play: Sports and the Problem of Masculinity.* Boston: Beacon Press.

Meyers, D. Tietjens. 2001. "The Rush to Motherhood—Pronatalist Discourse and Women's Autonomy. *Signs* 26: 735–33.

Miller M. N., and A. J. Pumariega. 2001. "Culture and Eating Disorders: A Historical and Cross-Cultural Review." *Psychiatry* 64: 93–110.

Minkoff, H. 1995. "Pregnancy and HIV Infection." Pp. 173–88 in *HIV Infection in Women*, edited by H. Minkoff, J. A. DeHovitz, and A. Duerr. New York: Raven Press.

Minkoff, H., J. A. DeHovitz, and A. Duerr, editors. 1995. *HIV Infection in Women.* New York: Raven Press.

Minto, C., and S. Creighton. 2001. "Objective Cosmetic and Anatomical Outcomes at Adolescence of Feminising Surgery for Ambiguous Genitals done in Childhood." *Research Letter. Lancet* 358: 124–25.

Mishler, E. G. 1984. *The Discourse of Medicine: Dialectics of Medical Interviews.* Norwood, N.J.: Ablex.

————. 1981. "Viewpoint: Critical Perspectives on the Biomedical Model." Pp. 1–23 in *Social Contexts of Health, Illness, and Patient Care*, edited by E. G. Mishler et al. Cambridge: Cambridge University Press.

MMWR. 2001. *CDC Morbidity and Mortality Weekly Report* 50 (July 20): 599–603.

Moldow, G. 1987. *Women Doctors in Gilded-Age Washington: Race, Gender, and Professionalization*. Urbana and Chicago: University of Illinois Press.

Molitor, F., J. D. Ruiz, J. D. Klausner et al. 2000. "History of Forced Sex in Association with Drug Use and Sexual HIV Risk Behaviors, Infection with STDs and Diagnostic Medical Care: Results from the Young Women Survey." *Journal of Interpersonal Violence* 15: 262–78.

Montagu, A. 1974. *Coming into Being Among the Australian Aborigines*, 2d ed. London: Routledge.

Moore, L. J. 1997. "'It's Like You Use Pots and Pans to Cook. It's the Tool': The Technologies of Safer Sex." *Science, Technology & Human Values* 22: 434–71.

Moore, L. J., and A. E. Clarke. 1995. "Clitoral Conventions and Transgressions: Graphic Representations of Female Genital Anatomy, c1900–1991." *Feminist Studies*. 21: 255–301.

————. 2001. "The Traffic in Cyberanatomies: Sex/Sexuality/Gender in Local and Global Formations." *Body & Society* 7: 57–96.

Morantz-Sanchez, R. M. 1985. *Sympathy and Science: Women Physicians in American Medicine*. New York: Oxford University Press.

Morris, J. 1993. "Feminism and Disability." *Feminist Review* 43: 57–70.

Mosca, L., P. Collins, D. M. Herrington et al. 2001. "Hormone Replacement Therapy and Cardiovascular Disease." *Circulation* 104: 499–503.

Moynihan, C. 1998. "Theories in Health Care and Research: Theories of Masculinity." *BMJ* 317: 1072–75.

Muller, C. 1990. *Health Care and Gender*. New York: Russell Sage.

Muncy, R. 1991. *Creating a Female Dominion in American Reform, 1890–1935*. New York: Oxford University Press.

Murphy, R. F. 1990. *The Body Silent*. New York: Norton.

Nam, C. B., I. W. Eberstein, and L. C. Deeb. 1989. "Sudden Infant Death Syndrome as a Socially Determined Cause of Death." *Social Biology* 36: 1–8.

Nechas, E., and D. Foley. 1994. *Unequal Treatment: What You Don't Know about How Women Are Mistreated by the Medical Community*. New York: Simon and Schuster.

Neigus, A., S. R. Friedman, R. Curtis et al. 1994. "The Relevance of Drug Injectors' Social and Risk Networks for Understanding and Preventing HIV Infection." *Social Science and Medicine* 38: 67–78.

Nelson, J. L. 1998. "The Silence of the Bioethicists: Ethical and Political Aspects of Managing Gender Dysphoria." *Journal of Clinical Ethics* 9: 213–30.

Nicolette, J. D., and M. B. Jacobs. 2000. "Integration of Women's Health into an Internal Medicine Core Curriculum for Medical Students." *Academic Medicine* 75: 1061–65.

Nicolosi, A., M. Leite, M. Musico et al. 1994. "The Efficiency of Male-to-Female and Female-to-Male Transmission of the Human Immunodeficiency Virus: A Study of 730 Stable Couples." *Epidemiology* 5: 570–75.

Nnko, S., R. Washija, M. Urassa et al. 2001. "Dynamics of Male Circumcision Practices in Northwest Tanzania." *Sexually Transmitted Diseases* 28: 214–18.

Nonnemaker, L. 2000. "Women Physicians in Academic Medicine: New Insights from Cohort Studies." *New England Journal of Medicine* 342: 399–405.

Nosek, M. A., M. E. Young, D. H. Rintala et al. 1995. "Barriers to Reproductive Health Maintenance among Women with Physical Disabilities." *JWH* 4: 505–18.

Notzer, N., and S. Brown. 1995. "The Feminization of the Medical Profession in Israel." *Medical Education* 29: 377–81.

Novello, A. Coello. 1995. "Introduction: Women and AIDS." Pp. xi–xiv in *HIV Infection in Women*, edited by H. Minkoff, J. A. DeHovitz, and A. Duerr. New York: Raven Press.

Nsiah-Jefferson, L., and E. J. Hall. 1989. "Reproductive Technology: Perspectives and Implications for Low-income Women and Women of Color." Pp. 93–117 in Ratcliff.

Nyamathi, A., and R. Vasquez. 1989. "Impact of Poverty, Homelessness, and Drugs on Hispanic Women at Risk for HIV Infection." *Hispanic Journal of Behavioral Sciences* 11: 299–314.

Obermeyer, C. Mahklouf. 1999. "Female Genital Surgeries: The Known, the Unknown, and the Unknowable." *Medical Anthropology Quarterly* 13: 79–106.

O'Farrell, N., and M. Egger. 2000. "Circumcision in Men and the Prevention of HIV Infection: A 'Meta-analysis' Revisited." *International Journal of Sexually Transmitted Diseases and AIDS*, 11: 137–42.

O'Hanlan, K. A. 1995. "Lesbian Health and Homophobia: Perspectives for the Treating Obstetrician/Gynecologist." *Current Problems in Obstetrics, Gynecology and Fertility* 18: 94–133.

Olesen, V. L., and A. E. Clarke. 1999. "Resisting Closure, Embracing Uncertainties, Creating Agendas." Pp. 355–57 in *Revisioning Women, Health, and Healing: Feminist, Cultural, and Technoscience Perspectives*, edited by A. E. Clarke and V. L. Olesen. New York: Routledge.

Orden, S. R., K. Liu, K. J. Ruth et al. 1995. "Multiple Social Roles and Blood Pressure of Black and White Women: The CARDIA Study." *JWH* 4: 281–91.

Osmond, M. Withers, K. G. Wambach, D. Harrison et al. 1993. "The Multiple Jeopardy of Race, Class, and Gender for AIDS Risk among Women." *Gender & Society* 7: 99–120.

O'Sullivan, S., and P. Parmar. 1992. *Lesbians Talk (Safer) Sex*. London: Scarlet Press.

Ouellette, S. K. 1993. "Inquiries into Hardiness." Pp. 77–100 in *Handbook of Stress: Theoretical and Clinical Aspects*, 2d ed., edited by L. Goldberger and S. Breznitz. New York: Free Press.

Padian, N. S., L. Marquis, D. P. Francis et al. 1987. "Male-to-Female Transmission of Human Immunodeficiency Virus." *JAMA* 258: 788–90.

Padian, N. S., S. C. Shiboski, and N. P. Jewell. 1991. "Female-to-Male Transmission of Human Immunodeficiency Virus." *JAMA* 266: 1664–67.

Paige, K. Ericksen. 1978. "The Ritual of Circumcision" *Human Nature*, May 1978, pp. 40–48.

Paige, K. Ericksen, and J. M. Paige. 1981. *The Politics of Reproductive Ritual*. Berkeley: University of California Press.

Parker, R. C. 1992. "Sexual Diversity, Cultural Analysis, and AIDS Education in Brazil." Pp. 225–42 in Herdt and Lindenbaum.

Parlee, M. Brown. 1982a. "The Psychology of the Menstrual Cycle: Biological and Psychological Perspectives." Pp. 77–99 in *Behavior and the Menstrual Cycle*, edited by R. C. Friedman. New York: Marcel Dekker.

————. 1982b. "Changes in Moods and Activation Levels during the Menstrual Cycle in Experimentally Naive Subjects." *Psychology of Women Quarterly* 7: 119–31.

————. 1994. "The Social Construction of Premenstrual Syndrome: A Case Study of Scientific Discourse as Cultural Contestation." Pp. 91–107 in *The Good Body: Asceticism in Contemporary Culture,* edited by M. G. Winkler and L. B. Cole. New Haven, Conn.: Yale University Press.

Patton, C. 1990. *Inventing AIDS.* New York: Routledge.

————. 1994. *Last Served? Gendering the HIV Pandemic.* London: Taylor & Francis.

Pear, R. 2001. "Advocates for Patients Barged In, and the Federal Government Changed." *NYT,* June 5.

Peifer, D. 1999. "Seeing is Be(liev)ing." Pp. 31–34 in *Restricted Access: Lesbians on Disability,* edited by V. Brownworth and S. Raffo. Seattle, Wash.: Seal Press.

Perls T. T., and R. Fretts. 1998. "Why Women Live Longer than Men." *Scientific American Presents* 9(2): 100–3.

Peteren, M., and D. McNeil. 2001. "Maker Yielding Patent in Africa for AIDS Drug." *NYT,* March 15.

Phillips, D. P., and K. A. Feldman. 1973. "A Dip in Deaths before Ceremonial Occasions: Some New Relationships between Social Integration and Mortality." *American Sociological Review* 38: 678–96.

Phillips, D. P., and E. W. King. 1988. "Death Takes a Holiday: Mortality Surrounding Major Social Occasions." *Lancet* 337: 728–32.

Phillips, D. P., T. E. Ruth, and L. M. Wagner. 1993. "Psychology and Survival." *Lancet* 342: 1142–45.

Phillips, D. P., and D. G. Smith. 1990. "Postponement of Death until Symbolically Meaningful Occasions." *JAMA* 263: 1947–51.

Pierre-Pierre, G. 1996. "Man Who Helped Wife Die to Serve 6 Months." *NYT,* May 18.

Pies, C. 1995. "AIDS, Ethics, Reproductive Rights: No Easy Answers." Pp. 322–34 in *Women Resisting AIDS: Feminist Strategies of Empowerment,* edited by B. E. Schneider and N. E. Stoller. Philadelphia: Temple University Press.

Pincus, H. A., T. L. Tanielian, and S. C. Marcus et al. 1998. "Prescribing Trends in Psychotropic Medications: Primary Care, Psychiatry, and Other Medical Specialties." *JAMA* 279: 526–31.

Pinn, Vivian W. 2001. "Science and Advocacy as Partners: The Office of Research on Women's Health in the 1990s. *JAMWA* 56: 77–78.

Polych, C., and D. Sabo. 2000. "Sentence—Death by Lethal Infection: IV-Drug Use and Infectious Disease Transmission in North American Prisons." Pp. 173–83 in *Prison Masculinities,* edited by D. Sabo, T. Kupers, and W. London. Philadelphia: Temple University Press.

Pope, H., K. Phillips, and R. Olivardio. 2000. *The Adonis Complex* New York: Free Press.

Preves, S. E. 1998. "For the Sake of the Children: Destigmatizing Intersexuality." *Journal of Clinical Ethics:* 9: 411–20.

Pringle R. 1998. *Sex and Medicine: Gender, Power and Authority in the Medical Profession.* Cambridge: Cambridge University Press.

Prior, J. C., Y. M. Vigna, M. T. Schechter, and A. E. Burgess. 1990. "Spinal Bone Loss and Ovulatory Disturbances." *New England Journal of Medicine* 323: 1221–27.

Profet, M. 1993. "Menstruation as a Defense against Pathogens Transported by Sperm." *Quarterly Review of Biology* 68: 335–81.

Ptacek, J. 1988. "Why Do Men Batter Their Wives?" Pp. 133-57 in *Feminist Perspectives on Wife Abuse*, edited by K. Yllö and M. Bograd. Newbury Park, Calif.: Sage.

Quinn, P., and S. Keys Walsh. 1995. "Midlife Women with Disabilities: Another Challenge for Social Workers." *Affilia* 10: 235–54.

Rahman, A., and N. Toubia. 2000. *Female Genital Mutilation: A Guide to Laws and Policies Worldwide*. London: Zed Books.

Reid, P. Trotman. 2000. "Women, Ethnicity, and AIDS: What's Love Got to Do with It?" *Sex Roles* 42: 709–22.

Reisine, S. T., and J. Fifield. 1988. "Defining Disability for Women and the Problem of Unpaid Work." *Psychology of Women Quarterly* 12: 401–15.

Renteln, A. Dundes. 1992. "Sex Selection and Reproductive Freedom." *Women's Studies International Forum* 15: 405–26.

Reunanen, A. 1993. "Juhlan Aika Ja Tuonen Hetki" ("The Time of Celebration and the Time of Death"). *Duodecim* 109: 2098–103.

Reverby, S. M. 1987. *Ordered to Care: The Dilemma of American Nursing, 1850–1945.* Cambridge: Cambridge University Press.

Rhode, D. 2001. "A Health Danger from a Needle Becomes a Scourge Behind Bars." *NYT*, August 6.

Riessman, C. Kohler. 1998. "Women and Medicalization: A New Perspective." Pp. 46–63 in *The Politics of Women's Bodies: Sexuality, Appearance and Behavior*, edited by R. Weitz. New York: Oxford University Press.

Riska, E. 1993. "Introduction." Pp. 1–12 in *Gender, Work and Medicine: Women and the Medical Division of Labor*, edited by E. Riska and K. Wegar. Newbury Park, Calif.: Sage.

———. 2001. *Medical Careers and Feminist Agendas: American, Scandinavian, and Russian Women Physicians*. Hawthorne, N.Y.: Aldine de Gruyter.

———. 2002. "From Type A Man to the Hardy Man: Masculinity and Health." *Sociology of Health and Illness* 24: 347–58.

Riska, E., and K. Wegar. 1993a. "Women Physicians: A New Force in Medicine?" Pp. 76–93 in *Gender, Work and Medicine: Women and the Medical Division of Labor*, edited by E. Riska and K. Wegar. Newbury Park, Calif.: Sage.

———, editors. 1993b. *Gender, Work and Medicine: Women and the Medical Division of Labor*. Newbury Park, Calif.: Sage.

Rittenhouse, C. A. 1991. "The Emergence of Premenstrual Syndrome as a Social Problem." *Social Problems* 38: 412–25.

Robbins, C. A., and S. S. Martin. 1993. "Gender, Styles of Deviance, and Drinking Problems." *Journal of Health and Social Behavior* 34: 302–21.

Romito, P., and F. Hovelaque. 1987. "Changing Approaches in Women's Health: New Insights and New Pitfalls in Prenatal Preventive Care." *International Journal of Health Services* 17: 241–58.

Rossi, A. S., and P. E. Rossi. 1977. "Body Time and Social Time: Mood Patterns by Menstrual Cycle Phase and Day of the Week." *Social Science Research* 6: 273–308.

Roter, D. L., and J. A. Hall. 1998. "Why Physician Gender Matters in Shaping the Physician-Patient Relationship." *JWH* 7: 1093–97.

Roter, D., M. Lipkin, and A. Korsgaard. 1991. "Sex Differences in Patients' and Physicians' Communication during Primary Care Medical Visits." *Medical Care* 29: 1083–93.

Rothman, B. Katz. 1982. *In Labor: Women and Power in the Birthplace.* New York: Norton.

———. 1986. *The Tentative Pregnancy.* New York: Viking.

———. 1989. *Recreating Motherhood: Ideology and Technology in a Patriarchal Society.* New York: Norton.

Rousso, H. 1988. "Daughters with Disabilities: Defective Women or Minority Women?" Pp. 139–71 in *Women with Disabilities: Essays in Psychology, Culture, and Politics,* edited by M. Fine and A. Asch. Philadelphia: Temple University Press.

Ruzek, S. Burt. 1978. *The Women's Health Movement: Feminist Alternatives to Medical Control.* New York: Praeger.

Ruzek, S. Burt, and J. Becker. 1999. "The Women's Health Movement in the United States: From Grass-Roots Activism to Professional Agendas." *JAMWA* 54: 4–8, 40.

Sabo, D., and D. F. Gordon, editors. 1995. *Men's Health and Illness: Gender, Power and the Body.* Newbury Park, Calif.: Sage.

Sabo, D., K. Miller, M. Farrell et al. 1999. "High School Participation, Sexual Behavior, and Adolescent Pregnancy: A Regional Study." *Journal of Adolescent Health.* 25: 207–16.

Sachs, S. 2001. "Clinics' Pitch to Indian Émigrés: It's a Boy." *NYT,* August 15.

Sack, K. 2001. "AIDS Epidemic Takes Toll on Black Women." *NYT,* July 3.

Sandelowski, M. 1993. *With Child in Mind: Studies of the Personal Encounter with Infertility.* Philadelphia: University of Pennsylvania Press.

Santow, G. 1995. "Social Roles and Physical Health: The Case of Female Disadvantage in Poor Countries." *Social Science and Medicine* 40: 147–61.

Scheper-Hughes, N. 1994. "An Essay: 'AIDS and the Social Body.'" *Social Science and Medicine* 39: 991–1003.

Schneider, B. E., and N. E. Stoller, editors. 1995. *Women Resisting AIDS: Feminist Strategies of Empowerment.* Philadelphia: Temple University Press.

Schoen, E. J., T. E. Wiswell, and S. Moses. 2000. "New Policy on Circumcision— Cause For Concern." *Pediatrics* 105: 620–23.

Scully, Diana. 1994. *Men Who Control Women's Health: The Miseducation of Obstetrics and Gynecologists.* New York: Teachers College Press.

Scully, D., and P. Bart. 1973. "A Funny Thing Happened on the Way to the Orifice: Women in Gynecology Textbooks." *American Journal of Sociology* 78: 1045–50.

Seals, B. F., R. L. Sowell, A. S. Demi et al. 1995. "Falling through the Cracks: Social Service Concerns of Women Infected with HIV." *Qualitative Health Research* 5: 496–515.

Sexton, P. C. 1982. *The New Nightingales: Hospital Workers, Unions, New Women's Issues.* New York: Enquiry Press.

Shaul, S., P. J. Dowling, and B. F. Laden. 1985. "Like Other Women: Perspectives of Mothers with Physical Disabilities." Pp. 133–42 in *Women and Disability: The Double Handicap,* edited by M. J. Deegan and N. A. Brooks. New Brunswick, N.J.: Transaction Books.

Shell-Duncan, B. and Y. Hermlund, editors. 2000. *Female "Circumcision" in Africa: Culture, Controversy, and Change.* Boulder Colo.: Lynne Reinner.

Shilling, C. 1993. *The Body and Social Theory.* Newbury Park, Calif.: Sage.

Shilts, R. 1987. *And the Band Played On: People, Politics and the AIDS Crisis.* Baltimore, Md.: Penguin.

Shweder, R. A. 2000. "What about "Female Genital Mutilation"? And Why Understanding Culture Matters in the First Place." *Daedalus* 129(Fall): 209–32.

Siegel-Itzkovich, J. 2000. "Baby's Penis Reattached After Botched Circumcision." *BMJ* 321: 529.

Simmons, R. G., S. Klein Marine, and R. L. Simmons. 1987. *Gift of Life: The Effect of Organ Transplantation on Individual, Family, and Societal Dynamics.* New Brunswick, N.J.: Transaction.

Simpson, B. J., and A. Williams. 1993. "Caregiving: A Matriarchal Tradition Continues." Pp. 200–11 in Kurth.

Smedley, B. D., A. Y. Stith, and A. R. Nelson (eds.). 2002. *Unequal Treatment: Confronting Racial and Ethnic Disparities in Health Care.* Washington, D.C.: National Academy Press.

Solarz, A., editor. 1999. *Lesbian Health: Current Assessment and Directions for the Future.* Washington, D.C.: National Academy Press.

Solomon, D. N. 1961. "Ethnic and Class Differences among Hospitals as Contingencies in Medical Careers." *American Journal of Sociology* 61: 463–71.

Sontag, S. 1989. *Illness as Metaphor and AIDS and its Metaphors.* New York: Doubleday.

Sourbut, E. 1997. "Reproductive Technologies and Lesbian Parents." Pp. 142–61 in *Science and the Construction of Women,* edited by M. Maynard. London: UCL Press.

Spark, R. F. 1988. *The Infertile Male: The Clinician's Guide to Diagnosis and Treatment.* New York: Plenum.

Specter, Michael. 2001. "India's Plague." *The New Yorker,* December 17: 74–85.

Stage, S. 1979. *Female Complaints: Lydia Pinkham and the Business of Women's Medicine.* New York: Norton.

Staples, R. 1995. "Health among Afro-American Males." Pp. 121–38 in *Men's Health and Illness: Gender, Power and the Body,* edited by D. Sabo and D. F. Gordon. Newbury Park, Calif.: Sage.

Starr, P. 1982. *The Social Transformation of American Medicine.* New York: Basic.

Steinem, G. 1978. "If Men Could Menstruate." *MS. Magazine* (October): 110.

Stevens, P. E. 1996. "Lesbians and Doctors: Experiences of Solidarity and Domination in Health Care Settings." *Gender & Society* 10: 24–41.

Stone, D. A. 1984. *The Disabled State.* Philadelphia: Temple University Press.

Strauss, A., S. Fagerhaugh, B. Suczek et al. 1985. *The Social Organization of Medical Work.* Chicago: University of Chicago Press.

Sudha, S., and S. Irudaya Rajan. 1999. "Disadvantage in India 1981–1991: Sex Selective Abortion and Female Infanticide." *Development and Change: Special Issue on Gendered Poverty and Well-being* 30(3): 585–18.

Sundari, T. K. 1994. "The Untold Story: How the Health Care Systems in Developing Countries Contribute to Maternal Mortality." Pp. 173–90 in E. Fee and N. Krieger, eds., *Women's Health, Politics, and Power.* Amityville, N.Y.: Baywood.

Swan, S., and E. Elkin. 1999. "Declining Semen Quality: Can the Past Inform the Present?" *Bioessays* 21: 614–22.

Szabo, R., and R. V. Short. 2000. "How Does Male Circumcision Protect Against HIV Infection?" *BMJ* 320: 1592–94.

Taggart, L. A., S. L. McCammon, L. J. Allred et al. 1993. "Effect of Patient and Physician Gender on Prescriptions for Psychotropic Drugs." *JWH* 2: 353–57.

Tanner, J., and R. Cockerill. 1996. "Gender, Social Change, and the Professions: The Case of Pharmacy." *Sociological Forum* 11: 643–60.

Thomas, W. I., and D. Swaine Thomas. 1927. *The Child in America*. New York: Knopf.

Thomson, R. Garland. 1994. "Review Essay: Redrawing the Boundaries of Feminist Disability Studies." *Feminist Studies* 20: 583–95.

Todd, A. Dundas. 1989. *Intimate Adversaries: Cultural Conflict Between Doctors and Women Patients*. Philadelphia: University of Pennsylvania Press.

Treichler, P. A. 1992. "AIDS, HIV, and the Cultural Construction of Reality. Pp. 65–98, in G. Herdt and S. Lindenbaum, eds., *The Time of AIDS: Social Analysis, Theory, and Method*. Newbury Park, Calif.: Sage.

———. 1999. *How to Have a Theory in an Epidemic: Cultural Chronicles of AIDS*. Durham, N.C.: Duke University Press.

Turner, B. S. 1984. *The Body and Society: Explorations in Social Theory*. London: Basil Blackwell.

———. 1992. *Regulating Bodies: Essays in Medical Sociology*. New York: Routledge.

Turner, H. A., R. B. Hays, and T. J. Coates. 1993. "Determinants of Social Support among Gay Men: The Context of AIDS." *Social Problems* 34: 37–53.

Turner, S. S. 1999. "Intersex Identities: Locating New Intersections of Sex and Gender." *Gender & Society* 13: 457–79.

van der Kwaak, A. 1992. "Female Circumcision and Gender Identity: A Questionable Alliance?" *Social Science and Medicine* 35: 777–87.

Van Devanter, N., V. Gonzales, C. Merzel et al. 2002. "Effect of an STD/HIV Behavioral Intervention on Women's Use of the Female Condom." *American Journal of Public Health* 92: 109–15.

Van Hall, E. V., M. Verdel, and J. Van Der Velden. 1994. "'Perimenopausal' Complaints in Women and Men: A Comparative Study." *JWH* 3: 45–49.

Ventura, S. J. et al. 2000. "Trends in Pregnancy and Pregnancy Rates by Outcome: Estimates for the United States, 1976–96." *National Vital Health Statistics*. CDC Web site.

Verbrugge, L. M. 1989. "The Twain Meet: Empirical Explanations of Sex Differences in Health and Mortality." *Journal of Health and Social Behavior* 30: 282–304.

Vertinsky, P. 1990. *The Eternally Wounded Woman: Woman, Doctors and Exercise in the Late Nineteenth Century*. Manchester, U.K.: Manchester University Press.

Voda, A. M., M. Dinnerstein, and S. R. O'Donnell, editors. 1982. *Changing Perspectives on Menopause*. Austin: University of Texas Press.

Waitzkin, H. 1983. *The Second Sickness: Contradictions of Capitalist Health Care*. New York: Free Press.

———. 1991. *The Politics of Medical Encounters: How Patients and Doctors Deal with Social Problems*. New Haven, Conn.: Yale University Press.

Waldron, I. 1995. "Contributions of Changing Gender Differences in Behavior and Social Roles to Changing Gender Differences in Mortality." Pp. 22–45 in *Men's Health and Illness: Gender, Power and the Body*, edited by D. Sabo and D. F. Gordon. Newbury Park, Calif.: Sage.

Wallace, J. I., J. Downs, A. Ott et al. 1983. "T-Cell Ratios in New York City Prostitutes." Letter. *Lancet* (1/8 January): 58–59.

Wallis, L. 1994. "Why a Curriculum on Women's Health?" Pp. 13–26 in *Reframing Women's Health*, by A. J. Dan. Newbury Park, Calif.: Sage.

Walsh, C., L. A. Anderson, and K. Irwin. 2000. "The Silent Epidemic of *Chlamydia trachomatis:* The Urgent Need for Detection and Treatment in Women." *JWH* 9: 339–43.

Walsh, M. Roth. 1977. *"Doctors Wanted: No Women Need Apply" Sexual Barriers in the Medical Profession, 1835–1975.* New Haven, Conn.: Yale University Press.

Warshaw, C. 1996. "Domestic Violence: Changing Theory, Changing Practice." *JAMWA* 51: 87–91.

Wawer, M. J., C. Podhisita, U. Kanungsukkasem et al. 1996. "Origins and Working Conditions of Female Sex Workers in Thailand: Consequences of Social Context for HIV Transmission." *Social Science and Medicine* 42: 453–62.

Waxman, B. F. 1994. "Up Against Eugenics: Disabled Women's Challenge to Receive Reproductive Services." *Sexuality and Disability* 12: 155–69.

Weiss, H. A., M. A. Quigley, and R. J. Hayes. 2000. "Male Circumcision and Risk of HIV Infection in Sub-Saharan Africa: A Systematic Review and Meta-Analysis." *AIDS* 14(Oct. 20): 2361–70.

Weiss, M. 1994. *Conditional Love: Parental Relations toward Handicapped Children.* Westport, Conn.: Greenwood Press.

Weitz, R. 1996. *The Sociology of Health, Illness, and Health Care: A Critical Approach.* Belmont, Calif.: Wadsworth.

———, editor. 1998. *The Politics of Women's Bodies: Sexuality, Appearance and Behavior.* New York: Oxford University Press.

Wendell, S. 1992. "Toward a Feminist Theory of Disability." Pp. 63–81 in *Feminist Perspectives in Medical Ethics*, edited by H. Bequaert Holmes and L. M. Purdy. Bloomington: Indiana University Press.

———. 1996. *The Rejected Body: Feminist Philosophical Reflections on Disability.* New York: Routledge.

Wermuth, L., J. Ham, and R. L. Robbins. 1992. "Women Don't Wear Condoms: AIDS Risk Among Sexual Partners of IV Drug Users." Pp. 72–94 in J. Huber and B. E. Schneider, eds., *The Social Context of AIDS* (Newbury Park, Calif.: Sage).

West, C., and D. Zimmerman. 1987. "Doing Gender," *Gender & Society* 1: 125–51.

Whitmore, R., J. I. Wallace, D. Bloch et al. 1996. "HIV Testing Rates in New York City Streetwalkers Have Declined." Poster at XI International Conference on AIDS, Vancouver.

Williams, C. L. 1992. "The Glass Escalator: Hidden Advantages for Men in the 'Female' Professions." *Social Problems* 39: 253–67.

Williams, L., and T. Sobieszyzyk. 1997. "Attitudes Surrounding the Continuation of Female Circumcision in the Sudan: Passing the Tradition to the Next Generation." *Journal of Marriage and the Family* 59: 966–81.

Wilson, M., and M. Daly. 1985. "Competitiveness, Risk Taking, and Violence: The Young Male Syndrome." *Ethology and Sociobiology* 6: 59–73.

Wilson, R. 1966. *Feminine Forever.* New York: M. Evans.

Winter, B. 1994. "Women, the Law, and Cultural Relativism in France: The Case of Excision." *Signs* 19: 939–74.

Wizemann, T. M., and M. Pardue, editors. 2001. *Exploring the Biological Contributions to Human Health: Does Sex Matter?* Washington, D.C.: National Academy Press.

Wu, Z., and M. S. Pollard. 1998. "Social Support among Unmarried Childless Elderly Persons." *The Journals of Gerontology* 53B(6): S324–35.

Yankauskas, E. 1990. "Primary Female Syndromes: An Update." *New York State Journal of Medicine* 90: 295–302.

Yedidia, M. J., and J. Bickel 2001. "Why Aren't There More Women Leaders in Academic Medicine? The Views of Clinical Department Chairs." *Academic Medicine* 76: 453–65.

Ziegler, R. G. 1993. "Migration Patterns and Breast Cancer Risk in Asian-American Women." *Journal of the National Cancer Institute* 85: 1819–27.

Zack, B., and O. Grinstead. 2001. "Collaborative Research to Prevent HIV among Male Prison Inmates and their Female Partners." *Science to the Community: Prevention*. Center for AIDS Prevention Studies, University of California San Franciso Web site.

Zimmerman, D., et al. 2000. "Gender Disparity in Living Renal Transplant Donation." *American Journal of Kidney Diseases* 36: 534–40.

Zita, J. 1988. "The Premenstrual Syndrome: "Dis-easing" the Female Cycle." *Hypatia* 3: 77–99.

———. 1993. "Heresy in the Female Body: The Rhetorics of Menopause." Pp. 59–78 in *Menopause: A Midlife Passage,* edited by J. C. Callahan. Bloomington: Indiana University Press.

Zola, I. K. 1982a. *Missing Pieces: A Chronicle of Living with a Disability.* Philadelphia: Temple University Press.

———. 1982b. "Tell Me, Tell Me." Pp. 208–16 in *Ordinary Lives: Voices of Disability and Disease,* edited by I. K. Zola. Cambridge, Mass.: Apple-wood Books.

Zoske, J. 1998. "Male Circumcision: A Gender Perspective." *Journal of Men's Studies* 6: 189–208.

Zucker, K. J. 1999. "Intersexuality and Gender Identity Differentiation." *Annual Review of Sex Research* 10: 1–69.

INDEX

Numbers in italics refer to tables.

ABOUT THE AUTHORS

Judith Lorber is Professor Emerita of Sociology and Women's Studies at Brooklyn College and The Graduate School, City University of New York. She is the author of *Gender Inequality: Feminist Theories and Politics* (Roxbury 1998, 2nd edition 2001), *Gender and the Social Construction of Illness* (1st edition, Sage 1997), *Paradoxes of Gender* (Yale 1994), and *Women Physicians: Careers, Status, and Power* (Tavistock 1984), and co-editor of *Revisioning Gender* (Sage 1999) and *The Social Construction of Gender* (Sage 1991). She was founding editor of *Gender & Society*, the official publication of Sociologists for Women in Society, and was chair of the ASA Sex and Gender Section. She has received the ASA Jessie Bernard Career Award and held the Marie Jahoda International Visiting Professorship of Feminist Studies at Ruhr University, Bochum, Germany. She is currently working on a new book, *Breaking the Bowls: Gender Theory and Social Change* (Norton).

Lisa Jean Moore is Assistant Professor of Sociology at the College of Staten Island, City University of New York. A qualitative and feminist medical sociologist, her work investigates the social processes that create meanings about human bodies. She has authored several articles about the construction of safer sex, human genital anatomy, and human semen. She is currently working on a new book, *Sperm Tales: The Making of Masculinities* (Routledge).

Breinigsville, PA USA
05 November 2010

248725BV00002B/3/P

9 780759 102385